Why We Fall Sick:

The Unknown Epidemic On How Insulin
Resistance Drives the Epidemic of Most
Chronic Diseases, and how to Fight It.

By

Mark R. Dickson

Disclaimer

Table of Contents

Introduction

In a world where mystery shrouded health, a lone scientist embarked on a quest for answers, penning the chronicles of "Why We Fall Sick: Insulin Resistance." Driven by a relentless curiosity, he unraveled the clandestine dance between our bodies and the hidden saboteur within – insulin resistance. The story unfolded in the labyrinth of cellular whispers, where insulin's once harmonious commands became distorted echoes.

As the scientist delved deeper, a revelation emerged: the silent epidemic of insulin resistance lay at the root of most chronic diseases. Through the pages of his book, he painted a portrait of an intricate system where muscles withered and bones crumbled under the stealthy influence of this unseen adversary.

Amidst the scientific tapestry, the narrative wove in tales of resilience, of individuals who, armed with newfound knowledge, defied the shadows cast by insulin resistance. The book became a beacon, guiding readers through the uncharted territories of lifestyle choices and holistic health. In the pages of "Why We Fall Sick," the scientist not only unveiled the enigma but also sparked a revolution, challenging the conventional notions of illness and inspiring a journey toward a healthier, more informed existence.

Chapter 1:. Brief Overview of The Current State of Health and Rising Chronic Diseases

In the quiet corridors of contemporary health, a subtle but unmistakable shift is occurring. The symphony of well-being is increasingly punctuated by discordant notes—rising rates of chronic diseases that cast a looming shadow over our collective vitality. The current state of health paints a sobering portrait, revealing a landscape where chronic diseases have emerged as formidable adversaries, challenging the very essence of our well-being.

In this age of technological marvels and unprecedented access to information, it is paradoxical that our health, instead of flourishing, is besieged by a surge in chronic maladies. Once confined to the margins, chronic diseases have now moved to the forefront of public health concerns, rewriting the narrative of wellness with an unsettling urgency. Diabetes, heart disease, obesity, and their silent accomplice, insulin resistance, are no longer whispered murmurs but resonate as a collective roar, demanding our attention.

Consider the seemingly inconspicuous rise in type 2 diabetes, a condition that has evolved from a rare occurrence to a prevalent force shaping global health trajectories. The incidence of diabetes has not merely risen; it has skyrocketed, transforming from a localized concern to a pervasive global challenge. This escalation is not exclusive to diabetes; it is mirrored in the surge of cardiovascular diseases, obesity rates, and a host of other chronic afflictions that now dominate the spectrum of modern health issues.

One cannot help but ponder the factors contributing to this unprecedented surge in chronic diseases. Our modern lifestyle, marked by sedentary habits and dietary choices often skewed towards processed indulgence, is a culprit that cannot be ignored. Fast-paced lives, adorned with convenience, inadvertently pave the way for a slow but insidious encroachment of diseases rooted in metabolic dysfunction.

Insulin resistance emerges as a linchpin in this complex narrative, quietly weaving its web in the intricate tapestry of our physiological functions. Once dismissed as a niche concern, insulin resistance has emerged as a hidden epidemic, the proverbial elephant in the room, influencing the trajectory of numerous chronic diseases. It is the silent orchestrator, conducting a symphony of metabolic discord that reverberates through the corridors of diabetes, cardiovascular diseases, and obesity.

The rise of insulin resistance is emblematic of a profound shift in our relationship with food and lifestyle. In an era where convenience often trumps nutritional wisdom, our bodies bear the brunt of the choices we make. The modern diet, laden with refined sugars and processed foods, has become a double-edged sword, tantalizing our taste buds while eroding our metabolic resilience.

It is crucial to recognize that the surge in chronic diseases is not a random occurrence; it is a reflection of systemic imbalances. The human body, intricately designed for resilience, is now grappling with challenges that extend beyond its evolutionary repertoire. As we navigate the complexities of modern living, our bodies, in their wisdom, respond to the onslaught with metabolic adaptations that, over time, lead to insulin resistance—a harbinger of an impending health crisis.

The narrative of rising chronic diseases is not one of despair but an urgent call to action. It beckons us to reassess our relationship with food, redefine our engagement with physical activity, and reconsider the very fabric of our lifestyle. It challenges us to dismantle the scaffolding of convenience that supports our modern existence and rebuild a foundation rooted in the principles of health and vitality.

In this exploration of the current state of health, we are confronted with a reality that demands introspection and change. Chronic diseases are not an inevitable consequence of progress; they are a reflection of the choices we make individually and collectively. The path forward requires a recalibration of our priorities, a shift in perspective that places health at the forefront of our societal values.

Concept of insulin resistance and its prevalence

In the quiet corridors of our bodies, a subtle rebellion brews, often unnoticed until the echoes of its consequences reverberate through the chambers of our health. This silent insurgent goes by the name of insulin resistance, a concept that transcends mere biochemical intricacies to cast a formidable shadow over our well-being.

Insulin, a hormone secreted by the pancreas, is the unsung conductor of our metabolic orchestra. It orchestrates the harmonious dance between glucose and our cells, ensuring a steady supply of energy. Yet, in the face of modern lifestyles and dietary choices, this intricate ballet can falter, giving rise to insulin resistance.

Imagine insulin as a key unlocking the door to our cells, allowing glucose to enter and fuel our bodies. However, with the insidious onset of insulin resistance, this once-efficient key finds its lock changed. The cells, in a misguided act of defiance, no longer respond as readily, leaving excess glucose lingering in the bloodstream like uninvited guests overstaying their welcome.

This biological standoff triggers a cascade of events, setting the stage for a hidden epidemic that lurks at the core of most chronic diseases. Its prevalence is alarming, silently weaving its tendrils through the fabric of our health. Affecting not just a select few, insulin resistance has become a pervasive force, a modern-day malady quietly infiltrating millions of lives.

Statistics tell a tale of rising numbers, but behind each figure lies an individual narrative of health challenges. Insulin resistance is not discriminatory; it knocks on the doors of the lean and the overweight alike. It infiltrates the lives of the sedentary and the active, making its presence felt across age groups and ethnicities.

One might wonder, how does this subtle resistance gain a foothold in our bodies? The answer is often found in the choices we make, the foods we consume, and the sedentary patterns of our contemporary lives. Highly processed diets, saturated with sugars and refined carbohydrates, act as the unwitting architects of insulin resistance. Coupled with a lifestyle that often favors sitting over movement, this metabolic insurgent provides fertile ground to thrive.

However, the prevalence of insulin resistance is not confined to the realms of personal choices alone. It is a societal challenge, influenced by the very fabric of our modern environment. Stress, a constant companion in the fast-paced world we inhabit, contributes to the biochemical milieu fostering insulin resistance. Sleep, or rather the lack thereof, becomes an accomplice, disrupting the delicate balance of hormonal regulation.

As we grapple with the consequences of this hidden epidemic, it becomes imperative to recognize that insulin resistance is not a standalone foe. It is the puppeteer orchestrating a symphony of chronic diseases. Type 2 diabetes, once considered an affliction of the aged, now finds a younger audience, its rise paralleling the surge in insulin resistance. Cardiovascular diseases, often attributed to a combination of genetic factors and lifestyle choices, bear the fingerprints of insulin resistance in their pathology.

Obesity, a visible manifestation of metabolic imbalance, is intricately entwined with insulin resistance, forming a symbiotic relationship that perpetuates each other's existence. The link doesn't end here; insulin resistance extends its influence to conditions as diverse as cancer, polycystic ovary syndrome (PCOS), and even neurodegenerative disorders like Alzheimer's.

The impact of insulin resistance on overall health

In the intricate dance of human biology, few partners are as crucial as insulin. A master orchestrator, insulin plays a central role in regulating blood sugar, a choreography essential for our body's energy balance. However, when this elegant ballet goes awry, a silent saboteur emerges—insulin resistance. A seemingly innocuous term that conceals a cascade of consequences, insulin resistance silently undermines our overall health.

The Dance of Insulin and Its Betrayal

Picture insulin as the conductor of a grand symphony, guiding glucose into cells for energy production. In a healthy body, cells respond promptly to insulin's cues, absorbing glucose efficiently. Yet, in the presence of resistance, this harmony shatters. Cells, like stubborn musicians, begin to disregard the conductor's instructions, leaving glucose stranded in the bloodstream.

The consequences reverberate throughout the body. Elevated blood sugar levels become a common refrain, triggering a domino effect on organs and systems. Insulin resistance becomes the discordant note disrupting the once seamless melody of health.

A House Divided: The Impact on Metabolism

The initial impact manifests in the realm of metabolism, where insulin resistance wreaks havoc on the body's ability to convert food into energy. As cells barricade themselves against insulin's call, glucose accumulation intensifies, laying the foundation for metabolic syndrome. This house divided becomes a breeding ground for chronic diseases, a fertile soil where conditions like type 2 diabetes take root and flourish.

Cardiovascular Symphony: A Discordant Beat

Beyond metabolism, the cardiovascular system becomes a battleground. Insulin resistance fuels inflammation and oxidative stress, casting a dark shadow on the cardiovascular symphony. The once smooth rhythm of blood flow becomes erratic, paving the way for atherosclerosis—the hardening of arteries—an insidious consequence that elevates the risk of heart disease.

Weighty Matters: The Obesity Connection

In the grand theater of health, insulin resistance takes center stage in the drama of obesity. Its impact on fat cells is profound, turning them into stubborn hoarders, resistant to releasing stored energy. The scales tip, literally and metaphorically, as weight accumulates. This association between insulin resistance and obesity becomes a dual-headed monster, each feeding off the other, contributing to a cycle of deteriorating health.

Cognitive Dissonance: Insulin Resistance and the Brain

As we navigate the labyrinth of health, the impact of insulin resistance extends to the enigmatic realm of the brain. Recent research suggests a link between insulin resistance and cognitive decline, with Alzheimer's disease emerging as a potential consequence. The brain, intricately connected to the body's metabolic symphony, succumbs to the discord orchestrated by insulin resistance.

The Ripple Effect: Insulin Resistance and Inflammation

In the silent war waged within, inflammation emerges as a relentless foot soldier. Insulin resistance fans the flames, creating an environment where chronic inflammation becomes the norm rather than the exception.

Organs, once resilient, now bear the brunt of this inflammatory assault, setting the stage for a myriad of chronic diseases, from arthritis to cancer.

Lifestyle as a Conductor's Baton: A Symphony of Prevention

In this symphony of health, lifestyle emerges as the conductor's baton—a powerful tool to mitigate the impact of insulin resistance. Regular exercise, a diet rich in nutrient-dense foods, and adequate sleep become the virtuoso performers, countering the disruptive notes of insulin resistance. As we wield these instruments of prevention, the body's resilience is rekindled, pushing back against the encroaching threat.

The Unfinished Score: Looking to the Future

In the narrative of health, insulin resistance remains an unfinished score, waiting for interventions and breakthroughs to alter its trajectory. Researchers delve into the intricacies of this metabolic dance, seeking new ways to harmonize insulin's symphony and restore health.

In the shadow of insulin resistance, the overarching impact on overall health unfolds as a tale of interconnected systems, each chapter revealing the profound consequences of this silent saboteur.

Chapter 2: Understanding Insulin Resistance

In the intricate dance of physiology, insulin orchestrates the symphony of energy regulation. However, when discord arises, a disruptive tune emerges—Insulin Resistance. In the inner chambers of our cells, where glucose meets destiny, insulin's authority is challenged. This chapter delves into the enigma of insulin resistance, decoding the molecular ballet that ensues within our bodies.

Insulin, the maestro of metabolism, usually directs cells to absorb glucose, the elixir of vitality. Yet, a subtle rebellion transpires when cells turn a deaf ear to insulin's guidance. We unravel the complexities of this defiance—what triggers it and how it unfurls into a metabolic quagmire. As the veil lifts, we find insulin resistance not merely a binary state but a spectrum, a continuum of metabolic sensitivity.

Venturing into the labyrinth of biochemical intricacies, we explore the multifaceted factors sculpting insulin resistance: genetics, lifestyle, and the relentless march of time. As we navigate this landscape, we confront the intimate ties between insulin resistance and metabolic syndrome, painting a vivid picture of the broader health implications.

This chapter invites you to decipher the language of insulin and peer into the molecular crucible where metabolic destinies are shaped. It beckons you to comprehend the intricate interplay that transforms a harmonious metabolic symphony into a discordant melody, laying the groundwork for the profound insights that follow.

Insulin and its role in the body

Insulin, an unassuming yet pivotal hormone, orchestrates a delicate dance within the human body, choreographing the intricate ballet of blood glucose regulation. Nestled within the pancreas, insulin emerges as the maestro of metabolic harmony, a regulator par excellence. Its primary mission: is to usher glucose, the lifeblood of cellular energy, into the cells, thereby sustaining the symphony of life.

At its core, insulin is a peptide hormone, a biological envoy dispatched by the pancreas to maintain a balance as delicate as a tightrope walker navigating a precarious wire. Picture insulin as the key to a cellular lock. When blood glucose levels rise, triggered by the consumption of carbohydrates, insulin gracefully steps forward to unlock the cells' gates. This balletic interplay ensures that glucose, akin to a vital energy courier, is ushered into the cellular realms where it fuels the body's myriad functions.

The pancreas, nestled inconspicuously behind the stomach, is the clandestine producer of insulin. This organ's dual role as an endocrine and exocrine powerhouse allows it to manufacture and release insulin into the bloodstream while simultaneously secreting digestive enzymes. It's a testament to nature's ingenuity that this seemingly unremarkable organ plays a central role in maintaining the delicate equilibrium of the body's metabolic terrain.

Within the bloodstream, insulin emerges as a sentinel, poised to detect any deviations from the body's preferred glucose levels. Its surveillance is relentless, ensuring that glucose does not soar to perilous heights after a sumptuous meal or plummet to dangerously low levels during fasting. In response to elevated blood glucose levels, insulin orchestrates a well-coordinated ballet of cellular absorption, enabling tissues to store excess glucose as glycogen for later use.

Yet, insulin's role extends far beyond mere glucose regulation. It wears the hat of a metabolic multitasker, influencing the fate of fats and proteins within the body's complex tapestry. As a conductor guiding the metabolic orchestra, insulin not only facilitates glucose entry into cells but also curtails the breakdown of stored fats and promotes their storage—a crucial function in the context of energy balance and body composition.

The symphony of insulin's actions reverberates throughout the body's diverse tissues, shaping not only metabolic destiny but also influencing cellular growth and repair. Within muscle cells, insulin stimulates the synthesis of proteins, fostering growth and repair. Simultaneously, it inhibits protein degradation, ensuring that the cellular machinery remains finely tuned for optimal function.

The intricate interplay of insulin extends its influence to the liver, a metabolic nexus of profound significance. Here, insulin reigns as a regulator of gluconeogenesis, the process by which the liver synthesizes glucose. By tempering this hepatic output, insulin maintains glucose homeostasis, preventing a runaway cascade that could disturb the equilibrium of the entire metabolic symphony.

It is crucial to recognize that insulin's role transcends the immediate concerns of glucose regulation. Its presence, or absence, resonates in the broader context of health. The absence of insulin, as witnessed in conditions like type 1 diabetes, shatters the orchestration of metabolic harmony, propelling the body into a state of chaos where glucose accumulates unchecked, fueling a cascade of systemic complications.

Conversely, the overzealous production of insulin, as observed in insulin resistance, marks a different dissonance. Like a maestro attempting to conduct a rebellious orchestra, insulin struggles to prompt cells to heed its cues, resulting in elevated blood glucose levels and metabolic turmoil. This defiance, if left unchecked, sets the stage for a host of chronic diseases, echoing the profound impact of insulin on the body's intricate equilibrium.

In this grand ballet of metabolism, insulin emerges as a central protagonist, a hormone with far-reaching implications for health and well-being. Its role extends beyond the conventional narrative of glucose regulation, permeating the fabric of cellular function, growth, and repair. To understand insulin is to unravel the intricate threads that weave the tale of metabolic balance—an epic saga where this unassuming hormone plays a starring role.

How does Insulin develop?

In the labyrinth of the human body's intricate processes, insulin resistance emerges as a formidable adversary, often lurking in the shadows before unleashing its detrimental effects on health. To fathom its essence, one must embark on a journey through the intricate ballet of hormones and cells, where insulin, the orchestrator, plays a pivotal role.

Insulin, a hormone secreted by the pancreas, acts as the conductor of the metabolic symphony. Its primary mission: is to facilitate the entry of glucose into cells, fueling the body's energy needs. Picture a finely tuned lock-and-key mechanism, where insulin is the key that unlocks the door, allowing glucose to enter cells and power essential functions.

However, the tale takes a dark turn when the cells, bombarded by constant signals, begin to close their doors to insulin's persistent knocking. This defiance marks the genesis of insulin resistance, a condition where cells lose their receptivity to insulin, leaving glucose stranded in the bloodstream.

The development of insulin resistance is a complex narrative, woven by a myriad of genetic, environmental, and lifestyle factors. Genetics, like an unseen hand-shaping destiny, can predispose individuals to insulin resistance. Some are born with a genetic code that renders their cells less responsive to insulin, setting the stage for a potential health saga.

Yet, genetics merely sets the scene; lifestyle takes center stage. Sedentary living, like a corrosive force, erodes the body's sensitivity to insulin. A life devoid of physical activity engenders a cascade of events – muscles, the primary reservoirs for glucose, become resistant to insulin's pleas, and excess fat accumulates, creating a domino effect of metabolic imbalance.

Diet, the sustenance of life, paradoxically becomes a harbinger of insulin resistance when laden with excessive sugars and refined carbohydrates. The modern diet, often characterized by overindulgence in processed foods, bombards the body with a deluge of glucose, overwhelming the insulin response and gradually desensitizing cells to its presence.

Amidst this complex interplay, the specter of obesity looms large. Adipose tissue once considered a passive storage unit, emerges as an active player in the insulin resistance drama. As fat cells burgeon, they release inflammatory signals, creating a hostile environment that further dampens insulin sensitivity, perpetuating a vicious cycle.

The march of time, an inevitable force, also plays a hand in the evolution of insulin resistance. Aging, like a silent infiltrator, erodes the body's resilience to insulin. Cells, wearied by years of metabolic demands, gradually lose their ability to respond efficiently, paving the way for insulin resistance to stealthily entrench itself.

Environmental factors, akin to external influences shaping an artist's masterpiece, contribute to the tapestry of insulin resistance. Chronic stress, a ubiquitous companion in the modern era, releases a torrent of stress hormones, sabotaging insulin's efforts and pushing the body towards resistance. Sleep, a cornerstone of well-being, becomes a casualty in this intricate dance, with insufficient rest further exacerbating insulin resistance.

In this intricate ballet of genetics, lifestyle, and environmental factors, insulin resistance emerges as a silent but potent force, setting the stage for a myriad of chronic diseases. The journey from insulin sensitivity to resistance is gradual, often imperceptible, like the slow turning of seasons. Cells, once harmoniously responsive to insulin's cues, succumb to the relentless onslaught of modern living, morphing into resistant entities that disrupt the delicate balance of metabolic harmony.

In unraveling the enigma of insulin resistance, one peels back the layers of a complex narrative, where genetic predispositions dance with lifestyle choices, and environmental factors wield influence. It is a tale of interconnectedness, where the body's cells, once in perfect harmony, fall prey to the insidious whispers of resistance

Linking insulin resistance to metabolic syndrome

In the intricate ballet of our body's internal workings, insulin plays a pivotal role, orchestrating the delicate balance of blood sugar regulation. However, when this dance falters, a silent disruptor emerges - insulin resistance. Unbeknownst to many, this subtle adversary doesn't merely stop at unsettling the glucose equilibrium; it extends its influence, weaving a complex tapestry that connects with a more ominous partner - metabolic syndrome.

To comprehend the link between insulin resistance and metabolic syndrome, one must first appreciate the nuanced interplay within our body's metabolic orchestra. Picture insulin as the master conductor, directing glucose into cells to fuel their activities. Yet, when resistance sets in, cells become obstinate, refusing the maestro's instructions. Glucose accumulates in the bloodstream, and the symphony of metabolic harmony is disrupted.

Metabolic syndrome, a constellation of interconnected risk factors, emerges as a haunting consequence. A domino effect is triggered: insulin resistance begets metabolic syndrome, and the latter amplifies the former.

The central theme in this narrative is insulin's indispensable role in lipid regulation. As insulin resistance tightens its grip, the body's ability to process fats is compromised. Triglycerides soar, high-density lipoprotein (HDL) cholesterol falters, and low-density lipoprotein (LDL) cholesterol assumes a more sinister profile. The once well-choreographed ballet of lipids transforms into a discordant performance, setting the stage for cardiovascular complications.

However, this is not merely a cardiovascular saga. Insulin resistance takes center stage in metabolic syndrome by instigating a proinflammatory environment. It prompts the release of inflammatory molecules, infiltrating organs and tissues. The inflammation, a hallmark of metabolic syndrome, becomes the silent architect of systemic chaos, linking seemingly unrelated conditions.

The abdominal region becomes a battleground, bearing witness to insulin resistance's impact. Fat cells, particularly visceral adipose tissue, become a manufacturing hub for inflammatory agents. The result? A visceral landscape rife with inflammation sets the scene for insulin resistance to exacerbate metabolic syndrome's progression.

Beyond the immediate consequences, insulin resistance amplifies the body's penchant for oxidative stress. Like rust corroding a once sturdy structure, oxidative stress deteriorates cellular integrity. Proteins and lipids bear the brunt, and cellular function is compromised. Metabolic syndrome, fueled by this oxidative storm, morphs into a multi-organ symphony of dysfunction.

Amidst this biochemical turbulence, the liver assumes a central role. Insulin resistance signals the liver to overproduce glucose, flooding the bloodstream. The pancreas valiantly responds by secreting more insulin, perpetuating a futile cycle. The result is a surge in blood sugar levels, further entwining insulin resistance with the metabolic syndrome narrative.

While insulin resistance and metabolic syndrome share a symbiotic relationship, it's crucial to acknowledge the catalysts that propel this alliance. Sedentary lifestyles and diets rich in refined sugars and saturated fats emerge as co-conspirators. The modern pace of life, marked by convenience foods and sedentary routines, fans the flames of insulin resistance, propelling its unholy matrimony with metabolic syndrome.

In this intricate dance between insulin resistance and metabolic syndrome, genetics also plays a role, acting as the silent choreographer shaping individual susceptibility. Some individuals possess a genetic predisposition that makes them more vulnerable to insulin resistance's insidious charm, ultimately inviting metabolic syndrome into their physiological narrative.

In unraveling the enigma of insulin resistance and its connection to metabolic syndrome, it becomes evident that this is not a linear storyline. Instead, it's a tapestry interwoven with genetic predispositions, lifestyle choices, and the intricate biochemical dance of our body's internal orchestra.

Chapter 3: The Connection to Chronic Diseases

Unlocking the cryptic dance between insulin resistance and chronic diseases reveals a complex symphony within our very cells. In this chapter, we embark on a journey through the vast landscape of ailments, uncovering the intricate threads that tie insulin resistance to the fabric of our health.

Begin with the towering specter of type 2 diabetes, where insulin resistance's fingerprints are unmistakable—each surge of insulin met with a diminishing response, a metabolic echo reverberating through the corridors of the pancreas. Traverse the treacherous terrains of cardiovascular diseases, where the endothelial cells bear the burden of insulin resistance, setting the stage for atherosclerosis and heartache.

Pause to scrutinize the expansive role insulin resistance plays in the realm of obesity, not merely a consequence but an architect of adiposity. As we unravel the genetic seams connecting insulin resistance to Alzheimer's and the oncogenic mysteries, the shadows of chronic diseases dissipate, revealing a shared origin in the twisted ballet of insulin and cellular response.

This chapter beckons the reader into the heart of the hidden epidemic, offering a panoramic view of the domino effect that begins with insulin resistance, echoing through the corridors of the body and triggering a cascade of chronic diseases. It is a narrative of interconnectedness, where understanding the root cause becomes the compass guiding us toward a healthier, disease-resistant future.

Diabetes

In the intricate tapestry of our health, the thread that weaves together insulin resistance and type 2 diabetes stands out boldly, unraveling a story of interconnected complexities. To comprehend this narrative, we embark on a journey into the physiological labyrinth where the dance between insulin and resistance takes center stage.

At its essence, diabetes is not merely a condition; it's a reflection of a disrupted dialogue within our bodies. The lead protagonist in this drama is insulin, the silent orchestrator of metabolic harmony. Imagine insulin as the conductor of a symphony, directing glucose - the musical notes of our energy - into cells for fuel. Yet, when insulin resistance steals onto the scene, this symphony becomes discordant, setting the stage for the onset of type 2 diabetes.

Insulin resistance, the rogue player in our metabolic drama, can be envisioned as a stubborn lock, impervious to insulin's key. This resistance, often rooted in lifestyle factors like poor diet and sedentary habits, gradually renders our cells deaf to insulin's instructions. Consequently, glucose accumulates in the bloodstream, akin to a melody gone awry, disrupting the delicate balance of our internal rhythm.

The link between insulin resistance and type 2 diabetes is akin to a complex dance routine. Picture insulin as a graceful dancer twirling through the bloodstream, weaving its way to unlock cellular doors. However, with resistance as its partner, this dance becomes strained, a choreography of missteps that propels us toward diabetes.

As the dance intensifies, so does the risk of developing type 2 diabetes. The persistent resistance places an increasing burden on the pancreas, the organ responsible for insulin production. Like a dancer pushed to their limits, the pancreas works overtime to compensate for the resistance, secreting more insulin in a desperate attempt to maintain glycemic harmony. This hyperinsulinemia, while a valiant effort, is unsustainable and, over time, exhausts the pancreas, setting the stage for diabetes to make its grand entrance.

The intricacies of this dance are further underscored by the role of adipose tissue, our body's storage depot. In the presence of insulin resistance, adipose tissue becomes a key player, releasing inflammatory substances that contribute to insulin resistance and further fueling the progression toward type 2 diabetes. It's a cyclic interplay where each misstep propels us closer to the diabetic denouement.

Unlocking the mystery of this dance requires a nuanced understanding of the risk factors that choreograph its movements. Genetics can dictate our susceptibility, casting a shadow over the stage that insulin resistance eagerly exploits.

Yet, lifestyle choices are the dance partners that truly guide the rhythm of this performance. A diet rich in refined sugars and unhealthy fats, coupled with a sedentary lifestyle, sets the stage for insulin resistance to pirouette into the limelight.

Understanding the link between insulin resistance and type 2 diabetes is not a passive observation; it's an invitation to actively participate in rewriting the script. Lifestyle modifications emerge as the choreographers are capable of redirecting the dance toward a healthier finale. A diet abundant in whole foods, coupled with regular physical activity, serves as the choreographic framework that can reshape the narrative, reducing insulin resistance and mitigating the risk of type 2 diabetes.

In our exploration of this intricate dance, the significance of early detection cannot be understated. Regular screenings, blood glucose monitoring, and awareness of subtle symptoms are the watchmen ensuring that the dance does not spiral into a diabetic crescendo unnoticed. Knowledge empowers us to intervene, to alter the steps of this metabolic ballet before it leads us down the path of irreversible consequences.

As we delve into the pages of this metabolic tale, the dance between insulin resistance and type 2 diabetes becomes a vivid narrative of our collective health. It's a story where understanding the intricacies of this dance offers not only enlightenment but also the power to reclaim control over our metabolic destiny.

Cardiovascular Diseases

In the symphony of our bodies, the heart takes center stage, orchestrating the rhythm of life. Yet, behind the scenes, a silent dancer known as insulin resistance is performing intricate moves that, when misunderstood, can lead to the crescendo of cardiovascular diseases.

The Ballet of Blood Sugar
Picture your body as a grand theater, with glucose as the prima ballerina and insulin as her partner. In a harmonious dance, insulin escorts glucose into cells, ensuring energy production. However, when insulin resistance steps into the choreography, the dance becomes a disjointed ballet. Cells resist the graceful guidance of insulin, causing a surge in blood sugar levels.

The Domino Effect on Cardiovascular Health
Insulin resistance, the covert disruptor, triggers a cascade of events that unfurl within the delicate

chambers of the heart. Elevated blood sugar levels induce inflammation, turning the heart's once harmonious rhythm into a discordant melody. This inflammation contributes to the formation of atherosclerosis, the notorious precursor to heart disease.

Atherosclerosis: The Veiled Culprit

In this cardiovascular drama, atherosclerosis plays the role of the veiled culprit. Insulin resistance not only fuels the flames of inflammation but also alters lipid metabolism. It sets the stage for the deposition of cholesterol and other fatty substances within the arterial walls, constructing the notorious plaques characteristic of atherosclerosis.

As these plaques grow, they narrow the arteries, imposing a restrictive chokehold on the flow of blood. The heart, accustomed to an unbridled dance with vitality, now labors to pump blood through the constricted vessels. The stage is set for a potentially catastrophic performance.

Blood Pressure: The Throbbing Drumbeat

Enter high blood pressure, the throbbing drumbeat in this cardiovascular composition. Insulin resistance, with its domino effect on the arteries, contributes to hypertension. The narrowed vessels require greater force from the heart to propel blood, creating a relentless rhythm that strains the cardiovascular system. Over time, this rhythmic strain becomes a silent accomplice to heart disease.

The Menacing Trio: Insulin Resistance, Diabetes, and Heart Disease

In the labyrinth of cardiovascular health, insulin resistance is not a solitary performer but part of a menacing trio, joined by its allies—diabetes and heart disease. Insulin resistance often precedes type 2 diabetes, and both conditions share a disturbing affinity for fostering cardiovascular complications.

Diabetes intensifies the cardiovascular plot by further aggravating inflammation and oxidative stress. The intricate dance between insulin resistance and diabetes becomes a synchronized assault on the heart, increasing the risk of heart attacks, strokes, and other cardiovascular events.

The Roadmap to Resilience
In this dance between insulin resistance and heart disease, knowledge becomes our choreographer. Understanding the steps of this intricate ballet empowers us to rewrite the script, turning a potential tragedy into a tale of resilience.

Lifestyle choices emerge as the spotlight in this narrative. A diet that tames blood sugar spikes, regular physical activity that cultivates insulin sensitivity, and stress management that soothes the heart's rhythm—all become pivotal moves in our counter-dance against insulin resistance and its cardiovascular repercussions.

Obesity

In the intricate dance of our body's mechanisms, insulin plays a central role, orchestrating the delicate balance between energy intake and expenditure. Yet, when this symphony falters, a hidden culprit emerges: insulin resistance. This covert condition not only disrupts metabolic harmony but unfurls a cascade of consequences, chief among them being the relentless advance of obesity.

Defying Expectations: Insulin's Double-Edged Sword

Insulin, often viewed as the gatekeeper of glucose, regulates the influx of sugar into cells for energy production. However, in a paradoxical twist, it also has a dual role in fat storage. When cells develop resistance to insulin signals, the delicate equilibrium tips towards fat accumulation. Imagine a once efficient traffic cop now struggling to control the flow, allowing chaos to ensue. Similarly, insulin resistance permits an excessive influx of glucose into fat cells, leading to an unrelenting expansion of adipose tissue.

Adipose Expansion: A Cellular Symphony Gone Awry

The body, in its infinite wisdom, stores excess energy as fat, a survival mechanism harking back to times of scarcity. Yet, in the modern era of abundance, this protective mechanism becomes a double-edged sword. Insulin resistance intensifies this predicament, turning adipose tissue into an ever-expanding metropolis. As insulin loses its effectiveness, fat cells hoard energy, growing larger and more resistant to the body's signals to release stored energy.

The Vicious Cycle: Insulin Resistance and Weight Gain

Imagine insulin resistance as a domino, its fall setting off a chain reaction leading straight to weight gain. As insulin struggles to guide glucose into cells, the pancreas compensates by producing more insulin. This increased insulin load, in turn, further heightens resistance, perpetuating a vicious cycle. As the body grapples with this internal discord, the scale tips inexorably towards weight gain.

Beyond the Waistline: Insulin Resistance's Ripple Effect

Insulin resistance, however, is not confined to mere weight gain; it orchestrates a symphony of metabolic disarray. Elevated insulin levels not only foster fat accumulation but also trigger inflammation and hormonal imbalances. This hormonal chaos not only exacerbates insulin resistance but also prompts the body to store even more fat, intensifying the struggle against obesity.

The Silent Architect: Insulin Resistance's Stealthy Onset

Insidious in its nature, insulin resistance stealthily creeps into our lives, often preceding noticeable weight gain. This silent architect of obesity operates in the shadows, altering the body's metabolism long before its effects become overt. By the time the bulging waistline becomes evident, insulin resistance has woven its web, leaving individuals grappling not only with excess weight but also with an intricate metabolic puzzle.

Breaking the Chains: Strategies for Overcoming Insulin Resistance and Obesity
While the connection between insulin resistance and obesity may seem formidable, there's hope in unraveling this intricate tapestry. Lifestyle modifications take center stage, with emphasis on a balanced diet that minimizes processed sugars and refined carbohydrates. Exercise, the unsung hero, emerges as a potent tool in improving insulin sensitivity, helping to break the chains of resistance.

Cancer

Insulin resistance, often associated with diabetes and metabolic disorders, is a clandestine player in the complex symphony of chronic diseases. Beyond its notorious connection to diabetes, insulin resistance has surreptitiously woven its threads into the fabric of cancer, adding a sinister note to the narrative of health.

Picture this: insulin as the conductor orchestrating the body's energy orchestra. In a healthy symphony, cells respond harmoniously to insulin's cues, absorbing glucose for energy. However, in the insulin-resistant scenario, the cells, like rebellious musicians, turn a deaf ear to the conductor. The consequence is a discordant rhythm, a metabolic melody that not only resonates with diabetes but also sets the stage for the ominous entry of cancer.

Cancer, that elusive adversary, is not a singular entity but a diverse group of diseases characterized by uncontrolled cell growth. Insulin resistance, it turns out, is a silent puppeteer manipulating the strings of cell signaling and metabolism, pushing the body toward conditions ripe for cancer development.

At the heart of this intricate dance lies the insulin-like growth factor (IGF) system. Insulin, a hormone with multifaceted roles, shares signaling pathways with IGF. In insulin resistance, the balance between these hormonal partners is disrupted, fostering an environment conducive to the unbridled growth of cells. Picture a garden where the delicate dance of insulin and IGF, when disrupted, nurtures the proliferation of malignant blooms.

Insulin resistance not only fuels the growth of existing cancer cells but also plants the seeds for their inception. Elevated levels of insulin and IGF, the hallmark of insulin resistance, act as growth stimulants for cells, providing fertile soil for the initiation of cancer. It's like pouring fuel on the embers, sparking the flames of cellular chaos.

The link between insulin resistance and cancer is not confined to a single type; rather, it infiltrates various cancer landscapes. Breast cancer, prostate cancer, and colorectal cancer—all bear the insidious fingerprints of insulin resistance. Imagine it as a silent infiltrator, a shadowy accomplice in the realm of oncogenesis.

Moreover, insulin resistance plays a role in the survival and progression of cancer cells. The altered metabolic landscape in insulin resistance offers cancer cells a strategic advantage—like a cloak of invisibility allowing them to evade the body's defense mechanisms. It's a survival game where insulin resistance tilts the odds in favor of the relentless advance of cancer cells.

But how does insulin resistance maneuver this perilous journey towards cancer? One key player is inflammation, the storm within. Insulin resistance ignites the flames of chronic inflammation, creating an environment conducive to cancer development. It's akin to a turbulent sea where cancer cells ride the waves of inflammation, finding refuge in the chaos.

Furthermore, insulin resistance influences the delicate dance of hormones within the body, disrupting the intricate ballet that regulates cellular functions. This disruption extends beyond insulin and IGF, involving hormones like estrogen and testosterone. In this hormonal tangle, insulin resistance whispers its sinister cues, contributing to the hormonal imbalances that fuel certain cancers.

As we delve into the molecular dance of insulin resistance and cancer, it becomes evident that the narrative extends far beyond the simplicity of cause and effect. It's a nuanced interplay where cellular communication, growth signals, and metabolic pathways converge, creating a conducive milieu for cancer's clandestine activities.

In unraveling this complex relationship, a pressing question emerges: can we sever the ties between insulin resistance and cancer? Understanding this intricate dance provides a roadmap for intervention. Lifestyle modifications, dietary choices, and targeted therapies emerge as potential choreographers, disrupting the rhythm that leads to cancer's crescendo.

Insulin resistance, once seen solely through the lens of diabetes, reveals its broader implications as a conspirator in the intricate plot of cancer. In this dance of cellular fate, insulin resistance leaves an indelible mark, weaving its threads into the narrative of chronic diseases. The journey from insulin resistance to cancer is a convoluted one, a path paved with disrupted signaling, inflammatory storms, and altered metabolic landscapes.

Non-Alcoholic Fatty Liver Disease (NAFLD)

In the intricate web of human health, where one ailment often weaves its roots into another, the connection between insulin resistance and Non-Alcoholic Fatty Liver Disease (NAFLD) emerges as a critical plotline. It's a story of interwoven metabolic threads that, if left unchecked, can lead to a cascade of health issues.

Insulin's Crucial Role: The Conductor of Metabolic Symphony

Imagine insulin as the conductor of a metabolic orchestra. Its role is to guide glucose into cells for energy production. However, when resistance builds, it's akin to musicians ignoring the conductor's cues. Insulin resistance arises when cells become deaf to insulin's directives, leading to a surplus of glucose circulating in the bloodstream.

The Silent Intruder: Insulin Resistance's Stealthy Onset

Unbeknownst to many, this insulin resistance, this silent intruder, has a close relationship with NAFLD. Picture the liver as the meticulous custodian of metabolic harmony. When insulin resistance knocks on its door, the liver's ability to regulate fat metabolism falters. It's like an overwhelmed janitor trying to clean up a mess, but the garbage bins are overflowing faster than they can be emptied.

Building the NAFLD Tapestry: A Metabolic Mosaic

Enter Non-Alcoholic Fatty Liver Disease, a condition where the liver accumulates excess fat. It's the intricate weaving of metabolic dysfunction, a tapestry spun from the threads of insulin resistance. The surplus glucose in the bloodstream becomes a tempting building material for the liver, which, in its struggle to cope, converts it into fat. This excess fat begins to cloak the liver, creating a metabolic masterpiece of dysfunction and inflammation.

The Domino Effect: Inflammation and Beyond

As the liver succumbs to this metabolic chaos, inflammation becomes its companion. The inflamed liver, a battleground of molecular skirmishes, begins to affect neighboring tissues. It's a domino effect, impacting not just the liver's ability to function but also sending ripples throughout the body. This inflammatory milieu is the precursor to more severe conditions, paving the way for a host of chronic diseases.

Connecting the Dots: Insulin Resistance as the Culprit

Step back, and the big picture emerges – insulin resistance is the quiet but powerful orchestrator of this metabolic symphony gone awry. Its influence extends far beyond the realm of glucose regulation, infiltrating the delicate balance of lipid metabolism in the liver. NAFLD, once thought of as an isolated liver condition, reveals itself as a piece in the larger puzzle of insulin resistance's impact on systemic health.

Beyond the Liver: Systemic Implications
But the story doesn't end with the liver. Insulin resistance, having cast its shadow over hepatic function, now sets the stage for broader health implications. Cardiovascular complications, Type 2 diabetes, and other chronic diseases become inevitable characters in this narrative. It's a reminder that the body is an intricately connected ecosystem, and disturbances in one part reverberate throughout the entire system.

The Redemption Arc: Managing Insulin Resistance for Liver Health
In the face of this metabolic drama, there is hope. Strategies to manage insulin resistance emerge as the protagonist in the plot. Lifestyle modifications, centered around a balanced diet and regular physical activity, become the tools to disarm the insulin-resistant villain. By addressing the root cause, these interventions

offer a chance to rewrite the metabolic storyline and prevent the escalation of NAFLD into more severe health complications.

Insulin Resistance With Alzheimer's and More

In the intricate tapestry of our health, one thread often overlooked weaves through diverse chronic diseases: insulin resistance. The silent saboteur, insulin resistance stealthily infiltrates the body's metabolic orchestra, playing a discordant tune that resonates in unexpected ways. Among the myriad consequences, its insidious connection to Alzheimer's disease stands out as a particularly poignant revelation.

The Mind-Bending Connection: Insulin Resistance and Cognitive Decline
Traditionally confined to discussions of diabetes and cardiovascular issues, insulin resistance's involvement in cognitive decline, specifically Alzheimer's disease, is a revelation that has

shifted the paradigm of our understanding. The brain, once considered exempt from the insulin-resistance drama, is not an ivory tower impervious to metabolic perturbations.

Alzheimer's, that haunting specter stealing memories and eroding cognition, has been linked to insulin resistance through a series of compelling studies. This sinister interplay unfolds as insulin resistance compromises the brain's ability to utilize glucose effectively. The brain, voraciously dependent on glucose as its primary fuel, encounters a roadblock, hampering its intricate dance of cognition and memory formation.

The Blood-Brain Barrier Breached

Insulin resistance is not content merely to disturb glucose utilization. It also engineers a breach in the blood-brain barrier, the vigilant guardian protecting the brain from harmful substances. This breach allows inflammatory molecules to infiltrate the brain, triggering a cascade of events that amplify the risk of neurodegenerative diseases like Alzheimer's. It's a stealthy invasion, turning the once-secure fortress of the brain into a vulnerable target.

The Inflammatory Symphony
Inflammation, orchestrated by insulin resistance, emerges as a key player in the Alzheimer's narrative. A chronic state of low-grade inflammation, fueled by the body's misguided response to insulin resistance, creates a hostile environment for neurons. This persistent inflammation not only accelerates the progression of Alzheimer's but also lays the groundwork for a fertile landscape for other chronic diseases.

Beyond Alzheimer's: Insulin Resistance's Far-reaching Impact
While the association with Alzheimer's is striking, insulin resistance casts its shadow across a broader spectrum of chronic diseases. Cardiovascular diseases, another realm where insulin resistance is a notorious accomplice, share a common stage with Alzheimer's. The

vascular bedrock of our brains, essential for cognitive function, becomes compromised in the face of insulin resistance, offering a dual assault on both heart and mind.

The connection extends to obesity and type 2 diabetes, where insulin resistance is often the harbinger of these health maladies. The link becomes a web, connecting seemingly disparate chronic diseases under the common denominator of insulin resistance. The body, an intricate tapestry of interconnected systems, unravels when insulin resistance pulls at its threads.

Untangling the Web: Diet, Lifestyle, and Insulin Sensitivity

Understanding insulin resistance's contribution to Alzheimer's and other chronic diseases necessitates unraveling the lifestyle and dietary factors that fuel its insidious progression. A diet rich in processed sugars and saturated fats, coupled with sedentary habits, lays the groundwork for insulin resistance to take center stage.

Conversely, lifestyle interventions become the unsung heroes in the battle against insulin resistance. Regular physical activity, ample sleep, and stress management emerge as powerful tools to enhance insulin sensitivity, disrupting the progression of this metabolic menace.

The Road Ahead: Navigating the Landscape of Prevention

As we delve deeper into the intricate dance between insulin resistance and chronic diseases, prevention emerges as a beacon of hope. Early interventions, emphasizing lifestyle modifications and heightened awareness, hold the promise of stemming the tide of insulin resistance before it orchestrates the symphony of chronic diseases.

In this narrative of health and disease, insulin resistance emerges as a formidable antagonist, its tendrils entwined in the complex narratives of Alzheimer's, cardiovascular diseases, obesity, and beyond. Understanding this connection is not merely a matter of academic curiosity; it is a clarion call to action. The body's intricate tapestry, vulnerable to the stealthy infiltration of insulin resistance, beckons us to rewrite its story—one of resilience, awareness, and a collective commitment to untangle the threads of chronic disease at their root.

Kidney Health

In the intricate dance of physiological processes within our bodies, insulin plays a lead role, orchestrating the delicate balance of glucose regulation. However, when this equilibrium is disrupted, a shadowy accomplice emerges insulin resistance. Its fingerprints are found not only in the rise of diabetes and heart disease but also in the often-overlooked realm of kidney health.

Insulin Resistance Unveiled

Imagine insulin as the conductor of a symphony, guiding glucose into cells for energy. In the face of resistance, this symphony falters. Insulin, once an efficient conductor, struggles to usher glucose into cells, leaving an excess in the bloodstream. As glucose levels rise, so does the burden on various organs, including the kidneys.

The Silent Saboteur: Kidney Damage

The kidneys, those unassuming bean-shaped organs, are the unsung heroes of our internal filtration system. However, when insulin resistance takes center stage, it morphs into a silent saboteur, gradually compromising kidney function. Elevated blood glucose levels place an undue load on these organs, leading to a cascade of detrimental effects.

Glomerular Filtration Under Siege

Within the intricate network of the kidneys, glomeruli act as meticulous sieves, filtering waste products and excess fluids from the blood. Insulin resistance, akin to a relentless assailant, disrupts this filtration process. The glomeruli become inflamed and permeable, allowing proteins to slip through, a condition known as proteinuria. This intrusion strains the kidneys, setting the stage for chronic kidney disease.

The Hypertension Tango

Insulin resistance not only sabotages the filtration process but also invites another accomplice to the scene: hypertension. As insulin loses its grip on glucose regulation, blood pressure rises. The kidneys, attempting to maintain equilibrium, respond by retaining salt and water. This hypertensive tango further amplifies the strain on the delicate renal structures.

Inflammation: A Smoldering Menace

Picture inflammation as a smoldering fire, often unseen but relentless in its damage. Insulin resistance stokes this inflammatory fire within the kidneys. Chronic inflammation damages renal tissues, paving the way for fibrosis – the formation of scar tissue. Like a web, this scar tissue ensnares the once-efficient filtering units, impairing kidney function and hastening the progression of renal decline.

The Crossroads of Diabetes and Kidney Health

As insulin resistance frequently heralds the onset of type 2 diabetes, the kidneys find themselves at the crossroads of this metabolic conundrum.

The relentless elevation of blood glucose in diabetes becomes a formidable foe for kidney health. The kidneys, overwhelmed by the incessant sugar surge, endure oxidative stress, contributing to further damage.

Microalbuminuria: A Subtle Signal

In the intricate tale of insulin resistance and kidney health, microalbuminuria emerges as a subtle signal of impending trouble. This condition, characterized by the presence of small amounts of albumin in the urine, is an early marker of kidney dysfunction. Often overlooked, it serves as a harbinger of the insidious dance between insulin resistance and renal compromise.

Breaking the Chains: Strategies for Kidney Health

Yet, amid the gloom, there is a glimmer of hope. Lifestyle interventions, such as adopting a diet rich in whole foods and engaging in regular physical activity, can break the chains forged by insulin resistance. These strategies not only address the root cause but also alleviate the burden on the kidneys. By enhancing insulin sensitivity, they act as shields, fortifying the kidneys against the onslaught of chronic disease.

Insulin Resistance on Aging Skin, Muscles and Bones

Aging Skin:

In the intricate tapestry of human physiology, the threads of aging are woven with precision, each strand contributing to the intricate narrative of time's inexorable passage. Among these threads, insulin resistance emerges as a silent but profound player, influencing not only internal landscapes but also leaving its indelible mark on the skin, the external mirror reflecting the underlying health of the body.

The Dance of Insulin and Aging: A Molecular Waltz

At the cellular level, insulin is not merely the gatekeeper of glucose; it orchestrates a complex dance within the body's cells. Insulin resistance disrupts this choreography, setting off a cascade of events that resonate beyond the confines of metabolic pathways. As insulin loses its effectiveness, cells are deprived of the signals to absorb nutrients, triggering a cellular response that echoes with the tones of aging.

Collagen, Elastin, and the Symphony of Skin Health

Enter the skin, our body's largest organ, and a canvas that bears witness to the passage of time. Collagen and elastin, the architectural pillars of youthful skin, find themselves caught in the crossfire of insulin resistance. As insulin fails to regulate nutrient absorption, the production of collagen diminishes, and the once resilient fibers of the skin lose their vitality. Elastin, the spring-like protein responsible for skin elasticity, succumbs to disharmony, contributing to the sagging and wrinkles that mark the aging process.

Inflammation: The Unwanted Crescendo

Insulin resistance, like a discordant note in an otherwise harmonious symphony, gives rise to chronic inflammation. This inflammatory crescendo reverberates through the skin, manifesting as redness, puffiness, and a general loss of vibrancy. The delicate balance of antioxidants, crucial for protecting the skin against environmental stressors, is disrupted, leaving the skin more susceptible to damage from free radicals.

The Dark Stains of Insulin Resistance

Beyond the visible signs of aging, insulin resistance increases its presence in less obvious ways. Hyperpigmentation, those stubborn dark spots that defy the pursuit of an even complexion, finds its roots in disrupted insulin signaling. As insulin resistance disrupts the delicate equilibrium of hormones, melanin production becomes erratic, leaving behind a map of time etched in shades of brown.

The Radiance of Resilience: Nurturing Skin Health

Yet, within the realm of insulin resistance and aging skin, there exists a glimmer of hope. The narrative need not be one of irreversible decline. By addressing the root cause — insulin resistance — one can unveil the path to resilient skin health. Through dietary choices that foster insulin sensitivity, embracing an active lifestyle, and nurturing the body's internal harmony, the skin can regain its luster.

In this dance between insulin and aging skin, the melody need not be mournful. It is an invitation to understand the intricate interplay of molecular forces and to compose a symphony of health that resonates through the years, echoing the beauty of vitality even as time gracefully advances.

Muscles:

In the intricate tapestry of human health, muscles play a pivotal role, not only in facilitating movement but also in metabolic regulation. However, lurking within the shadows of our metabolic machinery is a silent saboteur – insulin resistance. Unveiling its impact on muscles reveals a complex interplay that extends beyond mere movement.

At its core, insulin resistance disrupts the delicate dance between insulin and muscle cells. Insulin, traditionally known for its role in glucose regulation, also acts as a key player in muscle metabolism. When resistance sets in, it's akin to a miscommunication, where the muscle cells become less responsive to insulin's directives. The consequence? Impaired glucose uptake by muscles, leads to elevated blood sugar levels – a hallmark of diabetes.

Beyond the glucose conundrum, insulin resistance inflicts a deeper wound on muscles. It orchestrates a symphony of molecular events that culminate in muscle protein breakdown and hinder the synthesis of new proteins. This dual assault not only compromises muscle strength but also impedes the body's ability to repair and regenerate muscle tissue. The result is a gradual erosion of muscle mass, a phenomenon ominously known as sarcopenia.

The irony lies in the paradoxical relationship between insulin resistance and obesity. While insulin resistance is often associated with excess body weight, it simultaneously contributes to the loss of lean muscle mass. This dual impact creates a precarious situation where an individual may grapple with obesity and muscle wasting concurrently, further exacerbating health risks.

As we delve deeper into the intricacies of insulin resistance and muscle health, the importance of lifestyle factors comes to the forefront. Regular physical activity emerges as a formidable ally in combating insulin resistance. Exercise not only enhances insulin sensitivity in muscles but also stimulates the production of myokines –

molecules secreted by muscle cells with anti-inflammatory properties. Thus, the relationship between muscles and insulin resistance is not a one-sided affair; it's a dynamic dialogue where physical activity holds the power to reshape the narrative.

In the journey to unravel the enigma of insulin resistance and muscles, nutrition also plays a pivotal role. Dietary patterns rich in refined sugars and saturated fats, often implicated in the development of insulin resistance, pose a dual threat to muscle health. They not only contribute to the insulin resistance milieu but also lack the essential nutrients required for muscle maintenance and repair. A holistic approach to nutrition, emphasizing whole foods and adequate protein intake, emerges as a cornerstone in preserving muscle integrity amidst the challenges of insulin resistance.

Insulin Resistance and Bone Health

While the impact of insulin resistance on muscles is increasingly acknowledged, its influence on another critical aspect of our anatomy remains in the shadows – our bones. In the intricate dance of metabolic regulation, bones play a multifaceted role beyond providing structural support. Insulin resistance, it appears, has a silent hand in disrupting this delicate equilibrium.

At the core of the bone-insulin resistance interplay lies a complex web of signaling pathways. Insulin, traditionally revered for its role in glucose regulation, is a multifunctional player in bone health. It stimulates the production of osteoblasts, the cells responsible for bone formation, while simultaneously inhibiting the activity of osteoclasts, which break down bone tissue. However, when insulin resistance infiltrates this system, the delicate balance is upset.

Insulin resistance not only compromises the formation of new bone but also tips the scales in favor of bone resorption. The result is a net loss of bone density, a phenomenon intricately linked to osteoporosis. This silent erosion of bone mass sets the stage for increased fracture risk, transforming insulin resistance into a silent accomplice in the realm of skeletal health.

As we navigate the labyrinth of insulin resistance and its impact on bones, the role of inflammation emerges as a key player. Insulin resistance is not merely a disruption of glucose metabolism; it's a state marked by chronic low-grade inflammation. This inflammatory milieu, when extended to bone tissue, further accelerates bone loss. The intricate cross-talk between insulin resistance, inflammation, and bone health underscores the need for a comprehensive approach to address the root causes rather than merely managing the symptoms.

Lifestyle factors, once again, emerge as influential architects in this narrative. Weight-bearing exercises, recognized for their role in maintaining bone density, become even more crucial in the context of insulin resistance. The symbiotic relationship between muscles and bones takes center stage, emphasizing the interconnectedness of our physiological systems.

In the realm of nutrition, the story continues. Adequate intake of essential nutrients, particularly calcium and vitamin D, becomes a non-negotiable component in preserving bone health amidst the challenges of insulin resistance. The holistic approach to managing insulin resistance extends its reach to encompass bone health, painting a picture where lifestyle modifications and nutritional strategies become the brushstrokes on the canvas of skeletal resilience.

In unraveling the intricate relationship between insulin resistance and bones, a nuanced understanding emerges. It's not merely a disruption of metabolic pathways; it's a subtle yet potent force that transcends organs and systems. As we navigate this uncharted territory, the shadows dissipate, revealing a complex interplay that demands our attention and prompts a reevaluation of conventional perspectives on health and disease

Chapter 4: Diagnosis and Treatment

In the realm of health, the intricate dance of diagnosis and treatment unveils itself as a nuanced choreography, particularly when navigating the labyrinth of insulin resistance. Diagnosis, akin to a skilled detective, demands a keen eye for subtle clues—blood glucose levels, fasting insulin, and metabolic markers. It's a meticulous unraveling of the body's silent protest against the tyranny of insulin dysregulation.

Treatment, on the other hand, is an art form; a symphony of dietary adjustments, tailored exercise regimens, and, when necessary, pharmaceutical interventions. The canvas is vast, acknowledging the uniqueness of each individual's metabolic composition. Dietary shifts embrace the power of low-glycemic foods, while exercise becomes a sculptor, chiseling away at insulin resistance's obdurate facade.

Yet, the narrative extends beyond the clinical realm. It's a tapestry—despite the caveat—woven with narratives of those who've harnessed the alchemy of lifestyle changes to reclaim their health. This chapter unravels the intricacies, demystifying the science, and offering a roadmap for those navigating the labyrinth of insulin resistance. It's a compass, guiding the reader through the diagnosis intricacies and treatment kaleidoscope with an understanding that health, like art, is a dynamic masterpiece.

How is insulin resistance diagnosed?

insulin resistance lurks as a silent saboteur, often weaving its detrimental effects before revealing its presence. Diagnosing this elusive foe requires a nuanced understanding and a careful unraveling of the body's intricate metabolic dance.

The Silent Onset

Insulin resistance is a stealthy adversary, its early stages often devoid of noticeable symptoms. The journey toward diagnosis often begins with an astute clinician who, armed with suspicion, dives into the patient's medical history. Predisposing factors, such as a family history of diabetes, obesity, or a sedentary lifestyle, raise the index of suspicion.

Blood Glucose Levels: The First Clue

The cornerstone of diagnosing insulin resistance lies in assessing blood glucose levels. Fasting blood glucose tests serve as the initial gauge, capturing the body's response to a period of abstinence from food. Elevated fasting glucose levels may indicate the early stages of insulin resistance, reflecting the body's struggle to regulate blood sugar efficiently.

The Intricacies of Oral Glucose Tolerance Test (OGTT)

For a more comprehensive insight, the Oral Glucose Tolerance Test (OGTT) takes center stage. This involves consuming a specific amount of glucose followed by periodic blood draws. The body's ability to manage the glucose influx reveals itself in a temporal narrative, offering a dynamic portrayal of insulin response. A sluggish reaction manifests as prolonged elevation in blood glucose, signaling potential insulin resistance.

Hemoglobin A1c: A Window into the Past

Hemoglobin A1c, a reliable marker reflecting average blood glucose levels over the preceding two to three months, adds another layer to the diagnostic tapestry. While not a direct measure of insulin resistance, elevated A1c levels indicate long-term dysregulation of blood sugar. It serves as a historical account, chronicling the metabolic journey of the patient.

Fasting Insulin Levels: Peering Behind the Curtain

Beyond glucose-centric assessments, delving into fasting insulin levels uncovers the intricacies of insulin resistance. Insulin, the orchestrator of glucose metabolism, becomes the protagonist in this examination. Elevated fasting insulin levels, even in the presence of normal glucose, unveil the early stages of insulin resistance—a covert anomaly not easily deciphered by routine blood glucose tests alone.

The Lipid Connection: Triglycerides and HDL Cholesterol

A panoramic view of metabolic health involves scrutinizing lipid profiles. Elevated triglycerides and reduced high-density lipoprotein (HDL) cholesterol often accompany insulin resistance. Triglycerides, the fat molecules circulating in the blood, exhibit a dance with insulin. Their elevated presence hints at the metabolic disharmony associated with insulin resistance, while low HDL cholesterol serves as a reflective shadow of the body's struggle against metabolic imbalances.

The Clinical Crystal Ball: Imaging Techniques

In some instances, clinicians turn to imaging techniques to unravel the complexity of insulin resistance. Magnetic Resonance Imaging (MRI) and Computed Tomography (CT) scans provide glimpses into the distribution of adipose tissue, shedding light on the body's propensity for fat storage—a trait often magnified in insulin-resistant individuals.

Connecting the Dots: Comprehensive Assessment

Diagnosing insulin resistance is not a one-size-fits-all endeavor; it demands a mosaic of clinical insights. The amalgamation of fasting glucose, OGTT, hemoglobin A1c, fasting insulin, and lipid profiles paint a comprehensive picture. A clinician, armed with this multidimensional view, can decipher the intricate dance of insulin and glucose within the body, identifying deviations from the norm that hint at the presence of insulin resistance.

Traditional and alternative treatment approaches

Picture this: your body is a well-coordinated orchestra, with insulin playing the role of the conductor. But what happens when the maestro loses control, and chaos ensues? Welcome to the realm of insulin resistance, a sneaky culprit at the heart of many chronic diseases. Now, let's dive into the twin worlds of traditional and alternative treatments, the dynamic duo on a quest to restore harmony.

Traditional Treatments: The Pillars of the Medical Citadel

In the realm of traditional treatments, pharmaceuticals stand tall. Medications like metformin take center stage, aiming to enhance insulin sensitivity and keep blood sugar levels in check. It's like sending in the cavalry to rescue a besieged castle. But wait, there's more – thiazolidinediones, another set of defenders, work to reduce insulin resistance by targeting specific receptors.

Yet, the battlefield isn't just about medications. Lifestyle modifications play a crucial role. Imagine your daily routine as a mighty fortress; exercise, a formidable soldier, guards its walls, ensuring insulin does its job efficiently. And let's not forget the dietary archers, shooting down the enemies of insulin resistance with a diet rich in whole grains, fruits, and vegetables.

Monitoring blood sugar levels becomes the vigilant watchman, alerting you to any signs of trouble. Regular check-ups are like routine inspections, ensuring the fortress remains impervious to the lurking threat of insulin resistance.

Alternative Approaches: The Rebels with a Cause
Now, let's embark on a journey into the realm of alternative treatments. Picture it as a clandestine operation, a band of rebels challenging the established order. Enter acupuncture. Tiny needles punctuate the status quo, seeking to

restore the body's balance and improve insulin sensitivity. It's like a covert mission, silently dismantling the barriers erected by insulin resistance.

Not a fan of needles? Fear not, for yoga stands ready as the stealthy ninja, employing ancient postures and controlled breathing to vanquish insulin resistance. The mind-body connection becomes the secret weapon, an antidote to the stress that fuels insulin resistance.

Herbal remedies join the rebellion, with bitter melon and fenugreek playing pivotal roles. Nature's pharmacy provides an arsenal of weapons, each plant a potential antidote to insulin resistance.

The Blurring Lines: Integrative Approaches

But wait, what if we blend the best of both worlds? Enter integrative medicine, the peacemaker negotiating a truce between traditional and alternative approaches. Imagine a symphony where pharmaceuticals, acupuncture, and herbal remedies harmonize, working together to dismantle the fortress of insulin resistance.

Functional medicine, another player in this integrated saga, delves deep into the root causes. It's like Sherlock Holmes investigating the crime scene, seeking clues to unravel the mystery of insulin resistance.

Personalized nutrition steps onto the stage, acknowledging that one size does not fit all. Your body is unique, and so should be your approach to battling insulin resistance. It's like having a tailor-made suit, crafted to fit your individual needs.

The Road Less Traveled: Patient Narratives
Now, let's turn to the unsung heroes – the patients. Stories abound of individuals who've waged war against insulin resistance and emerged victorious. Sarah, once a prisoner of processed foods, embraced a whole-food diet and bid adieu to insulin resistance. John, a

devout yogi, found solace on the mat, his insulin sensitivity thriving with each sun salutation.

These narratives weave a tapestry of hope, proving that the battle against insulin resistance is not insurmountable. Each victory is a beacon, lighting the way for others on the same journey.

In this intricate dance between tradition and alternative, where insulin resistance is the puppeteer, the stage is set for a grand performance. Whether you choose the tried-and-true methods of traditional medicine, venture into the uncharted territories of alternative approaches, or find harmony in an integrated strategy, the goal remains clear – reclaiming your body's symphony from the clutches of insulin resistance

Medications and their role in managing insulin resistance

Managing insulin resistance can be a bit like navigating a busy city - you need the right tools and strategies to keep things moving smoothly. One crucial tool in this urban health landscape is medications. These tiny powerhouses can play a significant role in taming the insulin-resistant beast and helping you get back on the road to good health.

1. The Ins and Outs of Medications

Let's start with the basics. Medications for insulin resistance work in various ways, each with its superhero strength. Some boost insulin sensitivity, essentially teaching your body to listen more carefully when insulin says, "Hey, open the gates, we've got glucose to deliver!" Others help the pancreas produce more insulin, increasing the workforce to handle the glucose load.

2. Metformin: The Trailblazer

Imagine Metformin as the wise old guide in this journey. It's been around for ages and is often the first medication prescribed. Metformin doesn't just throw a party for insulin; it also helps the body use insulin more effectively. It's like giving your insulin a megaphone - louder, clearer, and more efficient.

3. Sulfonylureas: The Team Players
Now, enter Sulfonylureas, the team players. These medications help the pancreas release more insulin. They're like the cheerleaders on the sidelines, shouting, "Go, insulin, go!" However, they might not be suitable for everyone and can cause low blood sugar, so it's essential to have a coach (read: doctor) who knows the game plan.

4. Thiazolidinediones: The Negotiators
Thiazolidinediones are the negotiators in this insulin resistance saga. They help your body's cells respond better to insulin's instructions. Think of them as the diplomats, smoothing out the communication between insulin and your cells so glucose delivery becomes a diplomatic success rather than a battleground.

5. GLP-1 Receptor Agonists: The Moderators
GLP-1 Receptor Agonists are the moderators at this health party. They slow down the rate at which your stomach empties, reducing the post-meal glucose surge. They're like the bouncers, keeping the glucose levels from getting too rowdy and causing chaos in your bloodstream.

6. DPP-4 Inhibitors: The Traffic Controllers
Meet DPP-4 Inhibitors, the traffic controllers. They prevent the breakdown of a hormone that stimulates insulin release. It's like having a well-regulated traffic system in your body, ensuring a smooth flow of insulin without unnecessary bottlenecks.

7. SGLT2 Inhibitors: The Excess Glucose Bouncers
SGLT2 Inhibitors are the excess glucose bouncers. They prevent your kidneys from reabsorbing glucose, letting it exit your body

through urine. It's like having a doorman at a party, escorting the unruly glucose out before it causes any trouble.

8. The Marvel of Combination Therapies

Sometimes, it takes a superhero team-up. Doctors might prescribe a combination of medications to tackle insulin resistance from different angles. It's like having the Avengers of medications, each playing a unique role in keeping your metabolic universe in check.

9. Sidekicks and Supervision: Navigating Medication Waters

Now, before you embark on this medication adventure, remember that every hero needs a sidekick. Your doctor is your sidekick in this journey, keeping a close eye on how your body responds to the medications. Regular check-ins and monitoring ensure that the chosen medications are indeed helping, and not causing any unintended side effects.

The Bottom Line

In the bustling metropolis of managing insulin resistance, medications are indispensable tools in your utility belt. They come in various shapes and sizes, each with its superpower to restore balance to your body's insulin dance. So, if you're facing the insulin resistance monster, fear not—medications are here to help you reclaim your health and enjoy the vibrant city of well-being. Just remember, consult your healthcare superhero to find the perfect mix for your unique health journey

Chapter 5: Lifestyle and Dietary Factors

Alright, imagine your body is like a finely tuned car. Lifestyle and dietary choices are the fuel and maintenance it needs to run smoothly. In this chapter, we're diving into the nuts and bolts of how what you eat and how you live can either rev up your engine or leave you stuck on the side of the road with a metaphorical flat tire called insulin resistance.

Think of exercise as the oil change for your body – it keeps everything running smoothly. But it's not just about pumping iron at the gym; a simple daily stroll or a dance party in your living room can make a big difference. Now, let's talk about the gas in your tank – your diet. We'll dissect the roles of carbs, fats, and proteins, giving you the lowdown on how they can either fuel your journey or send you careening off course.

Ever heard of the Mediterranean diet? It's like giving your car the premium fuel it craves. We'll explore practical tips for integrating these changes into your life because, let's face it, life is too short for bland salads. Plus, we'll spill the beans on how sleep and stress management are the unsung heroes of keeping your engine humming smoothly. So buckle up, and let's hit the road to understanding how your daily choices can determine if you're cruising on the highway of health or stuck in the traffic jam of chronic issues.

Impact of Exercise and Physical Activities on Insulin Resistance

Let's talk about something we all know we should do more exercise. I get it, sometimes it feels like an uphill battle against your Netflix queue or the gravitational pull of the couch. But here's the deal – when it comes to insulin resistance, exercise is like the superhero swooping in to save the day.

You've probably heard the term "insulin resistance" thrown around, and maybe it sounds a bit like medical jargon. But think of it like this: your body has this amazing communication system, and insulin is like the messenger, telling your cells to open up and let glucose in. Insulin resistance is when your cells start playing hard to get, ignoring the messenger's calls.

Now, let's bring in our superhero – exercise. When you get moving, whether it's a brisk walk, a dance party in your living room, or hitting the gym, your muscles need energy. And guess what? They don't take no for an answer. They become these little insulin whisperers, saying, "Hey, we need some glucose here!" It's like a team-building exercise for your cells.

But it's not just about the immediate need for energy. Regular exercise has this magical long-term effect on your body's sensitivity to insulin.

It's like giving your cells a crash course in effective communication. They learn to listen better, respond faster, and overall become more chill when insulin comes knocking.

Let's dive into the nitty-gritty. When you engage in aerobic exercise – you know, the kind that gets your heart pumping – your muscles start using glucose for energy. This process doesn't just happen while you're sweating it out; it has a lasting impact. Your muscles become more efficient at using insulin, kind of like upgrading from an old flip phone to the latest smartphone.

Resistance training is another player in this game. Lifting weights or doing bodyweight exercises not only makes you feel like a badass but also helps build muscle mass. And here's the kicker – muscles are like glucose vacuums. The more muscle you have, the more glucose you can suck up, keeping those blood sugar levels in check.

Now, I know life can be hectic. Between work, family, and the never-ending to-do list, finding time for exercise feels like a luxury. But let me tell you, it's a necessity, especially if you're battling insulin resistance. Even if it's just a 20-minute dance party in your kitchen, it counts.

And don't think you need to become a gym rat overnight. Start small, find something you enjoy, and build from there. Whether it's a daily stroll, a weekend hike, or a game of pickup basketball, every bit adds up. Consistency is key, my friend.

Oh, and let's not forget about the stress-busting benefits of exercise. Stress and insulin resistance? They're like frenemies, and we want to break up that toxic relationship. Exercise helps your body manage stress more effectively, indirectly giving insulin a smoother ride through your system.

Now, I get it if you're thinking, "But I hate exercising!" Trust me, you're not alone. The key is to find something that doesn't feel like a chore. Maybe it's a dance class, gardening, or even chasing your dog around the backyard. Make it fun, make it yours.

Think of exercise as a way to show your body some love. It's not punishment for what you ate or a guilt trip for not hitting the gym yesterday. It's a celebration of what your body can do and an investment in its future health.

So, the next time you're contemplating another Netflix marathon, consider this: your body is a powerhouse, and exercise is the secret sauce to keep everything running smoothly. It's not about perfection; it's about progress. Lace-up those sneakers, hit the pavement, and let your body do its insulin dance. You won't regret it.

Role of Carbohydrates, Fats, and Proteins

Ever felt like your body's playing a trick on you? One day you're on top of the world, and the next, you're crashing harder than a failed rocket launch. Welcome to the mysterious world of insulin resistance, where what you eat can feel like a game of nutritional Russian roulette. Let's unravel the secrets behind the role of carbohydrates, fats, and proteins in this blood sugar tango.

Carbohydrates: The Good, the Bad, and the Misunderstood

Carbs get a bad rap, don't they? Picture them as the misunderstood rockstars of your diet. There are two types: simple and complex. Simple carbs, found in sugar-laden treats, can send your blood sugar on a rollercoaster ride, triggering insulin resistance. But complex carbs, the real MVPs found in fruits, veggies, and whole grains, are like the wise Gandalfs, guiding your body to balanced glucose levels. Choose your carbs wisely, my friend.

Fats: Not All Villains Wear Capes

Now, let's talk about fats. They're not the bad guys here. In fact, they play a crucial role in maintaining your insulin sensitivity. Healthy fats from avocados, nuts, and olive oil are like the unsung heroes of your diet. They help your cells absorb insulin better, ensuring it doesn't have to scream like an ignored GPS. Skip the trans fats and embrace the good ones – your cells will thank you.

Proteins: The Building Blocks of Resilience
Proteins, the muscle-makers, are not just for gym buffs. They're the building blocks of resilience against insulin resistance. Lean proteins like chicken, fish, and legumes keep you fuller for longer, preventing those blood sugar rollercoaster rides. Picture proteins as the construction workers in your body, building a strong foundation that insulin resistance can't easily shake.

The Tricky Trio's Dance with Insulin Resistance
Now, let's throw these three into the dance floor of insulin resistance. Carbs, when abused, can overwhelm your system, leading to insulin resistance. But, when paired with their trusty

sidekicks – healthy fats and proteins – they can create a harmonious symphony.

Imagine your plate as a canvas. The more colors you add, the more vibrant your health portrait becomes. Opt for a rainbow of veggies, a scoop of quinoa, a dollop of olive oil, and a side of grilled chicken. It's not just a meal; it's a nutritional masterpiece that keeps insulin resistance at bay.

Balancing Act: A Nutritional Cirque du Soleil
Balance is the name of the game. Too many carbs without their protein and fat buddies can lead to insulin resistance crashing your party. Conversely, too few carbs, and your body might start rationing insulin like it's in a wartime thriller.

Here's a hack: Pair high-fiber carbs with a sprinkle of healthy fats and a dash of proteins. It's like crafting a culinary love potion that tells insulin resistance to take a back seat. Your body will thank you with stable energy levels and a metabolism that purrs like a content cat.

The Tale of the Insulin Sensitivity Superheroes
When carbs, fats, and proteins work in harmony, they become the superhero squad maintaining order. Carbs are the citizens, fats are the infrastructure, and proteins are the law enforcers. Insulin resistance? It's the villain the superheroes keep at bay.

So, next time you're crafting your plate, think of it as casting for a blockbuster movie – carbs, fats, and proteins are the lead actors, and insulin resistance is the antagonist they're determined to defeat. Choose your cast wisely, and watch your body's epic saga unfold.

Mediterranean Diet and Other Approaches

Ever wondered if your kitchen could be the battleground against insulin resistance? Well, meet the Mediterranean diet, the unsung hero in the fight against the sneaky culprit behind many chronic diseases.

Picture this: a table filled with vibrant vegetables, olives, a splash of olive oil, and the aroma of herbs dancing in the air. That, my friend, is the Mediterranean diet—a celebration of fresh, wholesome foods inspired by the sunny shores of Greece, Italy, and Spain.

So, what's the fuss about? Let's dig into the science (without the lab coat, of course) and explore how this diet and other lifestyle approaches can kick insulin resistance to the curb.

The Mediterranean Love Affair with Health:
First things first, the Mediterranean diet isn't just a diet; it's a lifestyle. It's not about deprivation; it's about savoring the goodness Mother Nature provides. At its core, it champions plant-based foods: fruits, vegetables, nuts, and whole grains. Think of it as inviting the colors of the rainbow

to your plate—each hue bringing a unique set of nutrients and antioxidants.

But what makes it a heavyweight champion against insulin resistance? It's the healthy fats, my friend. Olive oil, a staple in this diet, isn't just a pretty face in the kitchen; it's a superhero combating inflammation and boosting insulin sensitivity. Healthy fats don't just sound good; they do good.

Say Yes to the Good Stuff:
Now, let's talk about the 'good stuff'—you know, the stuff that makes your taste buds do a happy dance. Fatty fish like salmon and mackerel are not just delectable; they're loaded with omega-3 fatty acids that keep inflammation in check. And those nuts and seeds? They're not just crunchy; they're packed with fiber and nutrients that regulate blood sugar levels.

And here's a secret ingredient: herbs. Not just for flavor, but for their anti-inflammatory powers. Rosemary, thyme, and oregano aren't just aromatic; they're on a mission to calm the insulin resistance storm.

A Dash of Lifestyle Changes:
Now, let's sprinkle some lifestyle magic into the mix. Lace up those sneakers; it's time to move. Exercise isn't just about fitting into those jeans; it's a dance party for your cells, making them more responsive to insulin. Even a leisurely stroll after dinner can make a difference.

And don't underestimate the power of shut-eye. Sleep isn't just for the weak; it's when your body works its repair magic. Skimping on sleep? That's a direct invitation to insulin resistance. So, let those Zs roll in like a welcome red carpet.

Beyond the Mediterranean:
But hey, the Mediterranean diet doesn't have a monopoly on goodness. Low-carb diets, like the trendy keto, can also be insulin-resistance warriors. By slashing those refined carbs, you tell insulin, "Hey, take a break. We got this."

Intermittent fasting, the rebellious cousin of traditional eating patterns, is another player in this game. It's not about starving yourself; it's about giving your body a break from constant fueling, allowing it to become more efficient in handling insulin.

The Nudge Towards a Healthier You:
In the grand scheme of things, there's no one-size-fits-all approach. It's about finding what clicks with you. Maybe it's the Mediterranean vibe, or perhaps you're more of a low-carb maestro. The key is making it a lifestyle, not a fleeting fling.

So, here's the deal: insulin resistance is a stealthy foe, but you've got an arsenal of fresh veggies, healthy fats, and lifestyle changes. It's not about a restrictive regimen; it's about embracing the foods and habits that love your body back.

Ready for the challenge? The kitchen is your battlefield, and your fork is your sword. Let's make every meal a victory in the fight against insulin resistance.

Sleep's Influence on Insulin Resistance

Have you ever wondered why getting a good night's sleep feels like hitting the reset button for your body? Well, let's dive into the fascinating world of sleep and discover how it plays a crucial role in something you might not expect: insulin resistance.

Imagine your body as a well-choreographed dance, with insulin as the lead dancer. Insulin's job is to help glucose (the energy from food) get into your cells so they can do their thing. Now, enter the troublemaker: insulin resistance. It's like a stubborn bouncer at the cell's door, making it harder for glucose to get in and party. And guess what disrupts this delicate dance routine? Yep, you guessed it – lack of sleep.

Picture this: you've had a rough night, tossing and turning, maybe binge-watching your favorite show. The next day, your body is groggy, and so is insulin. Studies show that even a single night of poor sleep can lead to insulin resistance, making it more challenging for glucose to enter your cells and provide the energy they need.

But why does this happen? Well, blame it on the hormonal havoc. Sleep is like a backstage manager, coordinating the release of hormones, and when you mess with that schedule, things go haywire. Cortisol, the stress hormone, takes the spotlight when you're sleep-deprived. Elevated cortisol levels contribute to insulin resistance, making it a tag team that disrupts the smooth operation of glucose entering your cells.

Now, let's talk about the rebel hormone: ghrelin. When you're sleep-deprived, ghrelin kicks into overdrive, making you feel hungrier than usual. It's like your body's way of seeking a quick energy fix after a night of incomplete rest. The problem is, that this often leads to poor food choices and overeating, putting an extra burden on insulin and making it work even harder to manage glucose.

But here's the kicker – it's not just about the quantity of sleep; quality matters too. Ever had a night of what you thought was good sleep but woke up feeling more tired than when you went to bed? That's the importance of deep, restorative sleep. It's during these precious hours that your body undergoes repair and regeneration, including insulin sensitivity.

Think of it this way: good sleep is like a superhero cape for your insulin. It helps restore its superpowers, ensuring it can efficiently usher glucose into your cells the next day. On the flip side, consistently poor sleep is like kryptonite, weakening insulin's ability to do its job and increasing the risk of insulin resistance.

Now, let's bust a common myth. It's not just the night owls who are at risk. Even if you're getting the recommended 7-9 hours of sleep, a misaligned sleep schedule – like irregular bedtimes – can throw off your body's internal clock, impacting insulin sensitivity.

But hey, it's not all doom and gloom. Improving your sleep habits can be a game-changer. Begin with a regular sleep schedule; your body craves routine. Make your sleeping environment cool, dark, and quiet. And put that phone away; the blue light emitted messes with your body's production of melatonin, the sleep hormone.

Now, let's talk about napping – the underrated hero. Short naps, around 20-30 minutes, can enhance alertness and performance without interfering with nighttime sleep. Just don't overdo it; we're aiming for a catnap, not a siesta.

In the grand scheme of things, treating your body to the sleep it deserves isn't just about feeling refreshed. It's about giving your insulin the support it needs to keep glucose in check and prevent the sneaky onset of insulin resistance.

So, next time you're tempted to sacrifice sleep for that late-night Netflix marathon, think twice. Your body, and your insulin, will thank you for a night of sweet dreams and a dance routine executed to perfection. After all, when it comes to insulin resistance, a well-rested body is a resilient body. Sleep tight!

Stress Reduction Techniques

Stress, we've all been there. The relentless deadlines, the never-ending to-do lists, the unexpected curveballs life throws at us - it's enough to make anyone's head spin. But here's the thing, beyond the frazzled nerves and sleepless nights, stress is also a silent culprit wreaking havoc inside our bodies. One of its sneakiest impacts? Insulin resistance.

Now, I know what you're thinking. Stress and insulin resistance? What's the connection? Well, buckle up, because it's a rollercoaster of hormones, emotions, and a dash of biology.

Picture this: you're stuck in traffic, running late for a meeting. Your palms are sweaty, your heart's racing and your brain is screaming at you. In this fight-or-flight mode, your body releases a flood of stress hormones, including the infamous cortisol. Now, cortisol isn't all bad; it helps you handle stress by releasing glucose into your bloodstream for quick energy. But here's where it gets tricky.

When stress becomes a constant companion, as it often does in our modern lives, cortisol keeps hanging around longer than it should. This prolonged exposure can lead to insulin resistance. You see, insulin, the superhero hormone, is responsible for ushering glucose into your cells. But when they're stressed out (pun intended), your cells start ignoring insulin's knocks, leaving glucose stranded in your bloodstream. Hello, high blood sugar levels and a potential one-way ticket to the diabetes town.

So, what's the antidote to this stress-induced insulin resistance drama? Stress reduction techniques, my friend. Let's dive into a few that could be your lifeboat in the turbulent sea of modern living.

1. Mindfulness Meditation:
Ever tried meditation? It's not just for the monks on the mountain; it's for us regular folks too. Mindfulness meditation is like a reset button for your stressed-out brain. Close your eyes, focus on your breath, and let the chaos in your mind settle. Studies show that regular mindfulness practice can help improve insulin sensitivity, giving cortisol a one-way ticket out of your system.

2. Yoga for the Win:
Not everyone can twist themselves into a pretzel, and that's okay. Yoga comes in all shapes and sizes. From gentle stretches to heart-pounding

flows, find what works for you. The beauty of yoga lies in its ability to combine movement, breath, and a sprinkle of zen. It's like a mini-vacation for your mind and bonus, it helps regulate those pesky stress hormones.

3. Laughter Therapy:

Yes, you heard it right. Laughter isn't just good for the soul; it's a stress-busting superhero. Watch a comedy, attend a live show, or simply gather with friends who crack you up. Laughter triggers the release of endorphins, your body's natural mood lifters. And guess what? Endorphins have a knack for calming stress hormones and, you guessed it, improving insulin sensitivity.

4. Nature's Embrace:

Step away from the screens, my friend, and take a nature break. Whether it's a stroll in the park, a hike in the woods, or just sitting by the beach, nature has a magical way of dialing down stress levels. The fresh air, the sound of birds chirping, the feel of grass beneath your feet – it's a prescription straight from Mother Nature herself.

5. Dance Like Nobody's Watching:
Cue the music and dance away your stress. Whether you've got the moves like Jagger or you're more of a two-left-feet kind of person, it doesn't matter. Dancing releases endorphins reduces cortisol, and, you guessed it, helps combat insulin resistance.

6. Sweat It Out Exercise for the Win
Exercise is like a superhero for your body, and when it comes to stress, it's a game-changer. You don't need a marathon on your schedule; a brisk walk, a dance session in your living room, or some yoga can do the trick. Exercise not only burns off stress but also improves insulin sensitivity, making it a double win.

7. Nature's Therapy: Embrace the Outdoors
There's something magical about nature. Trees, birds, and a gentle breeze – they have a way of calming the chaos within. Take a break from the

concrete jungle; even a short stroll in the park can work wonders.

8. Tech Detox: Unplug to Recharge

We're all guilty of being glued to our screens, whether it's for work or mindless scrolling. But here's the catch – that digital glow might be stressing you out. Give yourself permission to unplug for a bit. Turn off the notifications, step away from the screen, and let your mind breathe. Your insulin will thank you.

9. Laugh it Off: The Best Medicine

Laughter truly is the best medicine, and it's a fantastic stress-buster. Watch a funny movie, go to a comedy show, or just reminisce about those inside jokes with friends. Laughter not only reduces stress hormones but also triggers the release of feel-good endorphins. It's a natural stress antidote.

10. Conncct with Loved Ones: Your Support System

In the whirlwind of life, we often underestimate the power of human connection. Reach out to friends or family, share your day, or simply enjoy a good conversation. A strong support system can act as a shield against stress, creating a positive ripple effect on your insulin sensitivity.

11. Mind Your Plate: Stress-Busting Foods

Surprisingly, your diet plays a role in stress management. Opt for foods rich in omega-3 fatty acids, like salmon and walnuts, which have been linked to reduced stress levels. Dark chocolate in moderation can also be a delightful stress reliever – just one more reason to indulge guilt-free.

12. Sleep Soundly: Stress-Proof Your Nights

Ever noticed how stress can turn a good night's sleep into a distant dream? Prioritize your shut-eye. Create a bedtime routine, turn your bedroom into a haven of tranquility, and bid farewell to screens at least an hour before bedtime. Quality sleep not only rejuvenates you but also helps keep stress hormones in check.

Chapter 6: Lifestyle Interventions

Ever wondered if there's a secret code to crack the enigma of insulin resistance? Well, here it is: Lifestyle Interventions. It's not a fancy phrase for a crash diet or some extreme fitness routine; it's the real-life magic that can flip the script on insulin resistance and set you on a path to reclaiming your health.

Picture this: You, armed with the power of movement. Yeah, exercise – not the daunting marathon kind but the "let's take a stroll" variety. Walking, dancing, heck, even gardening – it all counts. Your body, soaking up the goodness of nutritious food like a sponge. No deprivation, just smart choices that make your taste buds do a happy dance.

But hold up, it's not just about what's on your plate or how many steps you clock. It's the zen zone – sleep. Imagine a world where bedtime isn't a battleground but a sanctuary. Stress? It becomes that annoying buzzing mosquito you swat away effortlessly.

Lifestyle Interventions is your superhero cape against insulin resistance. It's weaving simple, enjoyable habits into the fabric of your days. No rocket science, just everyday choices that nudge your body toward balance. So, grab that metaphorical cape, take a stroll, savor that salad, hit the sack with a smile, and bid adieu to the insulin resistance mystery. This chapter is your guide to making life the intervention your body has been silently pleading for.

Personalized Exercise Programs

Imagine your body as a finely tuned machine. Now, let's throw a wrench into the gears— Insulin Resistance. It's the sneaky troublemaker behind the curtain of many chronic diseases, making your body work harder than a toddler trying to fit a square block into a round hole. But fear not, because just as every superhero has a trusty sidekick, you have a powerful ally against insulin resistance: Personalized Exercise Programs.

First off, let's ditch the notion that exercise is a one-size-fits-all deal. It's more like a tailored suit, custom-made for your body's unique needs. The superhero costume of health, if you will. So, lace up those sneakers, and let's dive into the world of personalized exercise.

1. Know Thyself:
Before you start lifting weights or doing cartwheels (if you're into that), understand your current fitness level. No need to pull a hamstring on day one. Start slow, like a gentle jog rather than a sprint. Maybe even throw in a few power walks—your heart will thank you.

2. Mix It Up:
Variety is the spice of life, and it's the secret sauce for fighting insulin resistance. Your body thrives on diversity, so don't get stuck in a workout rut. Mix cardio, strength training, and

flexibility exercises. It's like a buffet for your muscles.

3. The Magic of Interval Training:
Let's talk about a workout style that's like the David Blaine of the exercise world—Interval Training. Short bursts of intense effort followed by rest periods can work wonders. It's like giving your metabolism a wake-up call, saying, "Hey, we've got work to do!"

4. Find Your Joyful Movement:
Exercising is part of what your body can do. Find an activity that brings you joy. Whether it's dancing like no one's watching, cycling through scenic routes, or practicing yoga in your living room—make it an experience, not a chore.

5. Strength Training:
Picture this: your muscles as bodyguards defending you against the chaos of insulin resistance. Strengthening exercises like weightlifting or resistance training build your muscle army, making them more insulin-

sensitive. You'll be a fortress against chronic diseases.

6. Team Up:

Everything's better with a buddy. Take a walk with a friend, family member, or even your pet. Having a workout partner not only makes training more enjoyable, but it also holds you accountable. It's like having your own cheer squad.

7. Pay Attention to Your Body:

Your body is your best friend, and it speaks to you. Take note of how you feel during and after exercise. Keep doing what you're doing if it's a joyful symphony. Adjust and see what works best for you if it's more like a creaky floorboard.

8. The Importance of Consistency:

Rome was not built in a day, and neither will your health journey. Consistency is the unsung hero in the battle against insulin resistance. Set realistic goals, stick to them, and watch the transformation unfold over time.

9. Make It a Lifestyle:

Let's shift the mindset. Exercise isn't a temporary fix; it's a lifelong commitment to your well-being. Integrate it into your daily routine, just like brushing your teeth. Soon, it'll be as natural as your morning cup of coffee.

10. Celebrate the Wins:

Whether it's running an extra mile, lifting a heavier weight, or simply sticking to your routine for a month—celebrate the wins, big and small. You're not just exercising; you're rewriting the script for a healthier, insulin-resistant-free future.

Tailored Dietary Plans

Picture this: your body is like a high-performance car, and insulin is the key to fueling it. When that key gets a bit rusty, things start to go haywire. That's where a tailored diet becomes your mechanic, fine-tuning your engine for optimal performance.

Understanding the Basics: Carbs, Fats, and Proteins

First off, let's talk about the three musketeers of nutrition: carbs, fats, and proteins. For someone dealing with insulin resistance, the goal is to keep these buddies in harmony. Think of them as a trio playing in a band – each instrument has a role, and they need to stay in sync.

Carbs – The Goldilocks Principle

Carbohydrates, often the misunderstood rockstars, come in two flavors: simple and complex. Simple carbs are like a sugar rush – quick and fleeting. Opt for complex carbs instead, the slow-release energy buddies found in whole grains, veggies, and legumes.

Fats – The Good, the Bad, and the Ugly

Now, onto fats – the James Bonds of nutrition. You want the good guys, the unsaturated fats, found in avocados, nuts, and olive oil. These fats are like secret agents, fighting inflammation and keeping your body in top-notch shape. Kick the trans fats and saturated fats to the curb – they're the villains causing trouble in your metabolic neighborhood.

Proteins – The Building Blocks

Proteins are the construction workers in this dietary masterpiece. They repair, build, and maintain. Fish, lean meats, tofu, and legumes are your protein-packed superheroes. They help keep you full, maintain muscle mass, and won't spike your blood sugar like a sugary snack.

The Mediterranean Love Affair

Ever dreamt of dining in the Mediterranean, basking in the sun, and savoring delicious, wholesome food? Well, good news – that dreamy diet is your ally against insulin resistance. Fruits, veggies, whole grains, fish, and olive oil – it's like a culinary vacation for your health.

Size Matters: Portion Control

Here's a little secret: portion control is the silent hero in this story. You don't need a math degree, just a bit of intuition. Your plate should be a colorful canvas – greens, a splash of protein, and a side of whole grains. It's like creating a masterpiece, but with food.

The Sneaky Culprits: Sugar and Processed Foods

Picture sugar as the villain in a blockbuster movie, causing chaos in your body. Cut down on sugary drinks, candies, and hidden sugars lurking in processed foods. Those sneaky culprits mess with your insulin sensitivity. Opt for the real deal – fruits for sweetness and whole foods over processed snacks.

The 80/20 Rule: Indulgence without Guilt

Let's be real – life without a treat now and then is just dull. Enter the 80/20 rule – make healthy choices 80% of the time, leaving a sweet 20% for indulgence. It's the guilt-free pass to enjoy that occasional slice of cake or a handful of chips.

Hydration – The Unsung Hero

Water is the unsung hero of the nutrition world. It's like the backstage crew, ensuring everything runs smoothly. Stay hydrated; it helps your cells do their job, including responding to insulin. Think of water as your body's personal cheerleader – always there, always cheering you on.

Experiment, Listen, and Learn

Creating a tailored diet is a bit like jazz – it's about improvisation. Experiment with different foods, listen to your body's rhythm and learn what works best for you. There's no one-size-fits-all. Maybe your body loves quinoa but throws a tantrum with too much pasta. Be the detective of your own health.

Behavioral Changes

Ever felt like your body is playing a game of hide-and-seek with its own insulin? You're not alone. Insulin resistance might sound like a complex term thrown around in medical circles, but let's break it down to simple, everyday language. It's like your cells putting up the "No Insulin Allowed" sign, and that can lead to a carnival of chronic diseases. But here's the secret weapon: behavioral changes. Yep, small tweaks in your daily habits can be the superhero cape your body needs to fight insulin resistance.

1. The Sneaky Dance of Sugar and Exercise
Picture this: your body as a dance floor, and insulin and sugar are partners in a not-so-fancy tango. When you're moving, grooving, and breaking a sweat, it's like the dance floor is alive with rhythm. Regular exercise is the ultimate DJ that keeps the insulin-sugar dance in sync. So, whether it's a salsa class, a jog in the park, or even a lively game of Twister, get your body moving – it's the coolest party in town.

2. Eating Habits: Ditch the Crash Diets for a Sustainable Love Affair with Food

Let's talk about food – the fuel that powers your body. Insulin resistance often gives a thumbs-down to refined carbs and sugars, but fear not, you don't have to bid farewell to your favorite treats. It's all about balance and moderation. Swap that sugar-loaded soda for a refreshing glass of water with a splash of lemon. Embrace whole foods like fruits, veggies, and whole grains – they're like the VIP pass to a healthier you.

3. Sleep: Your Body's Recharge Station

Imagine your body is a smartphone, and sleep is the charging cable. Without a full charge, your phone (or body) starts glitching. The same goes for insulin resistance. Lack of sleep messes with your body's insulin sensitivity, making it more resistant. So, tuck yourself in early, create a cozy sleep haven, and let your body recharge. It's like giving your superhero the rest it needs before another day of saving the world.

4. Stress: The Silent Enemy

Ever noticed how stress sneaks into your life like an uninvited guest? Well, it turns out that stress is like kryptonite for your insulin. It sends your body into a frenzy, making it resistant to insulin's superhero powers. Find your zen zone – be it yoga, meditation, or even a good belly laugh with friends. Your body will thank you, and insulin resistance won't stand a chance against your newfound calm.

5. Mindful Eating: Chew, Savor, Repeat

Eating isn't just about stuffing your face; it's a mindful experience. Slow down, savor each bite, and let your taste buds do the dance. This isn't just about enjoying your food – it's about giving your body time to register what's happening. When you eat mindfully, your body responds better to insulin. It's like creating a symphony of flavors that your body can appreciate and digest with ease.

6. Social Support: Your Insulin-Resistant Squad

No superhero tackles villains alone. Building a support squad is crucial in the fight against insulin resistance. Share your journey with friends, and family, or join online communities. When you have a team cheering you on, making behavioral changes becomes a group effort. Swap recipes, share victories, and turn your journey into a collective win against insulin resistance.

7. Small Wins: Celebrate Like You Just Saved the Day

Every step towards beating insulin resistance is a win, no matter how small. Celebrate these victories like you just conquered a dragon. Whether it's choosing a salad over fries or adding an extra lap to your evening walk, pat yourself on the back. Small changes add up, and before you know it, you'll be the hero of your own story, defeating insulin resistance one smart choice at a time.

Chapter 7: Research and Emerging Treatments

The landscape of health is shifting, and with it, our understanding of insulin resistance is evolving. But what's truly fascinating is the realm of research and the promising treatments that lie on the horizon. Picture this: a world where chronic diseases linked to insulin resistance are not just managed but potentially reversed. Let's dive into the cutting-edge science that's shaping this future.

Scientists are delving deep into the cellular intricacies of insulin resistance, seeking to unravel its mysteries. It's not just about identifying the problem; it's about understanding the very roots of it. Imagine researchers as detectives, peering into the inner workings of our cells to find the clues that unlock the secrets of insulin resistance.

One breakthrough avenue involves the role of inflammation. It turns out, chronic low-grade inflammation is like the silent accomplice in the insulin resistance saga. Researchers are exploring anti-inflammatory drugs, envisioning a day when we can not only manage but curb insulin resistance by addressing the inflammation that fuels it. It's like putting out the fire instead of just treating the smoke.

But here's where it gets even more exciting – personalized medicine. Imagine a healthcare plan tailored specifically for you, taking into account your genetic makeup, lifestyle, and the unique fingerprint of your insulin resistance. Scientists are exploring genetic therapies that could precisely target the roots of insulin resistance, offering a level of precision medicine that could transform the way we approach treatment.

Now, let's talk about the power of the gut. Yes, you heard it right – the gut microbiome.

Emerging research suggests that the trillions of microbes in our gut play a crucial role in regulating metabolism and insulin sensitivity. Probiotics and prebiotics could become powerful tools in the fight against insulin resistance, promoting a healthier balance of gut bacteria and potentially mitigating the risk of chronic diseases.

And there's more on the dietary front. Beyond just counting carbs, researchers are investigating the impact of specific nutrients on insulin sensitivity. Imagine a world where your plate isn't just a source of sustenance but a tool to combat insulin resistance. It's not just about what you eat but how it influences your body at the molecular level.

But let's not forget the role of technology. We're living in an era where our smartphones are smarter than ever, and researchers are harnessing this power for health. Mobile apps, wearables, and continuous glucose monitoring are not just gadgets; they're becoming integral tools in managing insulin resistance. Imagine having real-time insights into how your body responds to different foods, helping you make informed choices that directly impact your health.

Now, let's talk about the potential game-changer – regenerative medicine. The idea of repairing or replacing damaged tissues is no longer confined to the realms of science fiction. Stem cell therapies are being explored as a way to rejuvenate insulin-producing cells in the pancreas, offering hope for those grappling with diabetes and insulin resistance.

As we navigate this sea of possibilities, it's crucial to recognize the importance of ongoing research. The journey from a breakthrough in the lab to a transformative treatment for millions is a marathon, not a sprint. But with each discovery, we're getting closer to a future where insulin resistance is not just a puzzle to solve but a battle we can win.

So, here's to the scientists tirelessly working in labs, the individuals participating in clinical trials, and the hope that one day, the term "insulin resistance" won't be synonymous with chronic diseases but rather a challenge that we overcame together. The future is bright, and the possibilities are as vast as the universe itself. Stay curious, stay hopeful, and let's continue this journey into the unknown terrain of health and well-being.

The Role of Technology

In our fast-paced, tech-driven world, it's hard to escape the constant buzz of smartphones and the allure of the latest gadgets. But have you ever stopped to think about how technology is quietly playing a crucial role in the battle against insulin resistance and the myriad of chronic diseases it triggers? Let's dive into the digital frontier and explore the ways in which our tech-savvy tools are becoming unexpected heroes in the fight for better health.

First on the scene is the rise of wearable devices. You know, those nifty fitness trackers that adorn wrists like futuristic accessories. More than just counting steps, these little wonders are becoming health detectives. They monitor your heart rate, track your sleep patterns, and, yes, even gauge your glucose levels. It's like having a personal health assistant right on your arm, nudging you to move when you've been too sedentary, or giving you a gentle reminder that your body needs quality shut-eye.

But wearables are just the tip of the iceberg. Smartphone apps are stepping up to the plate, transforming our handheld devices into powerful allies against insulin resistance. Imagine an app that not only logs your meals but also analyzes their impact on your blood sugar. It's like having a nutritionist in your pocket, guiding you toward food choices that won't send your insulin levels on a rollercoaster ride. These apps provide real-time feedback, turning your daily decisions into informed choices that can positively influence your health.

Now, let's talk about the game-changer: telemedicine. The days of waiting in a sterile doctor's office are giving way to virtual consultations that happen in the comfort of your own home, thanks to video conferencing technology. For those managing insulin resistance, this means quicker access to healthcare professionals, personalized advice, and ongoing support—all without the hassle of a commute or the stress of navigating a crowded waiting room.

However, technology's impact on health goes beyond personal devices and virtual consultations. Big data is quietly revolutionizing the way we understand and tackle chronic diseases. Researchers are tapping into massive datasets to identify patterns, predict health trends, and develop targeted interventions. It's like having a crystal ball that reveals the future of healthcare—a future where precision medicine takes center stage, tailoring treatments to the individual based on their unique genetic makeup and lifestyle.

And let's not forget the role of social media in creating communities of support and shared experiences. Online platforms are connecting people from all corners of the globe who are dealing with insulin resistance. It's a virtual support group where struggles are shared, victories celebrated, and knowledge freely exchanged. The power of collective wisdom is facilitated by a few clicks and taps.

But perhaps the most exciting frontier in the tech-health alliance is the rise of artificial intelligence. Picture this: an AI-powered assistant that learns your habits, understands your body's responses, and offers personalized suggestions to keep insulin resistance at bay. It's like having a health-savvy sidekick, guiding you through the intricacies of daily living while adapting to your unique needs.

As we journey further into this tech-driven health landscape, one thing becomes clear: the role of technology in managing insulin resistance is not a mere subplot but a central theme. From wearables to telemedicine, big data to social networks, and AI to personalized apps, technology is weaving itself into the very fabric of our health narrative.

So, the next time you glance at your fitness tracker or input your meals into a health app, remember that you're not just engaging in a tech ritual—you're actively participating in a movement that's redefining how we approach and conquer the hidden epidemic of insulin resistance. It's a brave new world, where the tools in our hands are shaping the future of our well-being.

Conclusion

As we close the chapters on this journey through the labyrinth of insulin resistance and its insidious link to chronic diseases, let's talk about what really matters: you and your power to shape your health narrative. It's not about becoming a diet guru or a fitness fanatic overnight. It's about embracing the tiny triumphs and recognizing that every choice you make is a vote for the person you want to be, not just today, but for years to come.

Empowerment begins with understanding. In the quiet moments when you question that extra cookie or contemplate a brisk walk, remember this: your choices wield incredible influence over your health destiny. It's not about deprivation; it's about nourishment, not punishment. Your body is your lifelong companion, and the dialogue you share through food, movement, and rest can either be harmonious or discordant. You hold the pen, ready to write the next chapter.

No need for a grand transformation. Small, consistent steps create the most lasting change. Swap the elevator for the stairs, and choose a colorful plate of veggies over a monotone fast-food meal. Celebrate the vibrant, whole foods that fuel your body and mind. Invite friends for a stroll instead of a movie, transforming the mundane into the extraordinary.

Sleep is your unsung hero, a vital ally in this battle against insulin resistance. Prioritize it, cherish it, and watch your resilience soar. Stress, the silent saboteur, loses its grip when faced with laughter, mindfulness, and moments of stillness. You're not striving for perfection; you're embracing progress, letting go of guilt, and learning from missteps.

Remember, this journey isn't about reaching an elusive destination. It's about weaving health into the fabric of your life. Your body is an intricate masterpiece, and you are the curator. So, go ahead, and paint your canvas with choices that honor your well-being. You're not just fighting against illness; you're nurturing a flourishing existence. The power is in your hands. Seize it, savor it, and revel in the vitality that unfolds. Your health story awaits, and you are the storyteller.

Appendix

Glossary of Terms

Ever feel like you've landed in the middle of a medical drama where everyone's speaking a secret language? Fear not! Here's your backstage pass to the glossary, where we decode the perplexing terms surrounding insulin resistance:

Insulin:
The body's blood sugar maestro. Imagine insulin as the VIP ticket that lets glucose into your cells, ensuring they get the energy they need.

Insulin Resistance:
It's like a rebellious teenager slamming the door on their parent (insulin). Your cells resist insulin's charm, leading to elevated blood sugar levels. Cue the glucose rebellion!

Hemoglobin A1c:

Think of this as the diary of your blood sugar adventures. Hemoglobin A1c measures the average glucose levels over the past three months, giving you a sneak peek into your body's blood sugar history.

Non-Alcoholic Fatty Liver Disease (NAFLD):
Your liver's cry for help, signaling it's storing more fat than a bear preparing for winter. Contrary to the name, it has nothing to do with whiskey and everything to do with insulin resistance.

Mediterranean Diet:
Not your typical diet, but a lifestyle celebration of olive oil, vibrant veggies, fruits, and a cameo by fish. It's the culinary embodiment of "health is wealth."

OGTT (Oral Glucose Tolerance Test):
A medical rollercoaster where you gulp down a sugary concoction, and we watch how your blood sugar levels dance over time. It's the

ultimate test of your body's glucose management skills.

Adipose Tissue:
Fancy talk for body fat. It's not just insulation; it's a dynamic organ influencing hormones and playing a role in the intricate dance of insulin resistance.

Beta Cells:
The rockstars in your pancreas are responsible for producing insulin. They're the Beyoncé of the endocrine system.

Ketosis:
When your body shifts from carb-burning to fat-burning mode. It's like a metabolic makeover, popular in low-carb diets.

BMI (Body Mass Index):
The old-school scale for measuring whether you're a feather or a brick. While it has its critics, it's still a quick way to assess body weight in relation to height.

Microbiome:
The bustling community of microbes living in your gut. They influence everything from digestion to your body's response to insulin.

Polyunsaturated Fats:
The unsung heroes are found in foods like nuts, seeds, and fatty fish. They play a role in heart health and might have a cameo in insulin sensitivity.

Metabolic Syndrome:
A villainous squad of conditions, including high blood pressure, high blood sugar, excess body fat, and abnormal cholesterol levels. They team up to make life challenging but are often linked to insulin resistance.

Glucagon:
Insulin's partner in crime. While insulin ushers glucose into cells, glucagon encourages the liver to release glucose when energy is needed.

Additional Resources

So, you've reached the end of the book, but the journey toward understanding insulin resistance and reclaiming your health is just beginning. Here's a treasure trove of resources to keep you on the right track:

1. Websites:
American Diabetes Association

A hub of information on diabetes and insulin resistance, with resources for managing your health and lifestyle.
National Institute of Diabetes and Digestive and Kidney Diseases (NIDDK)

Your go-to for in-depth research and up-to-date information on diabetes and related conditions.

2. Books That Pack a Punch:
The Obesity Code by Dr. Jason Fung

Dr. Fung takes you on a journey through the complexities of obesity, including the role of insulin.
Good Calories, Bad Calories by Gary Taubes

A deep dive into the science of nutrition and how it affects our health, including insulin resistance.

3. Apps to Keep You Accountable:
MyFitnessPal

Track your meals, set fitness goals, and keep an eye on your nutrition with this user-friendly app.
Headspace

Managing stress is a crucial part of the insulin resistance battle. This app offers guided meditation and mindfulness exercises.

4. Community Support:
Reddit - r/diabetes

Join the conversation with real people sharing their experiences and insights on managing diabetes and insulin resistance.
Local Meetup Groups

Connect with people in your area facing similar health challenges. Sometimes, a cup of coffee and a shared story can be the best medicine.

5. Cooking Up Change:
Eat This Much

Generate meal plans that align with your nutritional needs, making healthy eating a breeze.

Cooking Light

Find delicious recipes that not only tantalize your taste buds but also keep insulin resistance in check.

Remember, knowledge is power, but action is the real game-changer. Use these resources to empower yourself on your journey to better health. Whether it's tweaking your diet, lacing up those sneakers, or finding support in unexpected places, you've got the tools to take charge. Here's to a healthier, happier you

Recipes and Meal plan

Hey there, health warriors! So, you've learned about the sneaky culprit—insulin resistance—and now you're itching to fight back with your secret weapon: food! Let's dive into some scrumptious recipes and a 7-day meal plan that'll make your taste buds dance while giving insulin resistance a run for its money.

Day 1: Fueling Your Day Right

Good morning! Let's kick off your journey to combat insulin resistance with a hearty breakfast. How about starting the day with a delicious spinach and feta omelet? It's packed with protein to keep you full and fueled. Pair it with a slice of whole-grain toast and a handful of berries for that extra antioxidant boost.

Lunch is all about a colorful salad loaded with veggies, grilled chicken, and a sprinkle of nuts.

The fiber from the veggies and the lean protein will keep your energy stable throughout the day.

Dinner tonight is a comforting bowl of salmon with quinoa and roasted vegetables. Salmon provides those omega-3 fatty acids that are fantastic for your heart, and quinoa gives you a dose of complex carbs without the blood sugar spikes.

Day 2: Mix It Up for Balance

Time for a quick and easy breakfast that's also rich in fiber and healthy fats. Greek yogurt with a handful of almonds and sliced strawberries – a tasty combo that satisfies your sweet tooth while supporting your health goals.

Lunch involves a turkey and avocado wrap using whole-grain tortillas. Turkey brings in lean protein, while avocados contribute heart-healthy monounsaturated fats. It's a portable and delicious option for those busy afternoons.

Dinner switches gears with a vegetarian stir-fry. Load up on colorful veggies like bell peppers, broccoli, and snap peas, and toss them with tofu for a plant-powered protein punch. Serve it over brown rice for a wholesome, satisfying meal.

Day 3: Embrace the Mediterranean Vibes

Mornings are brighter with a Mediterranean-style breakfast. Try a Greek yogurt parfait with layers of fresh fruit, granola, and a drizzle of honey. It's a delightful start that balances proteins, carbs, and natural sweetness.

For lunch, think Mediterranean salad with chickpeas, cherry tomatoes, cucumber, and feta. Dress it with olive oil and a squeeze of lemon for that classic Mediterranean flavor. Don't forget a serving of whole-grain crackers on the side.

Dinner introduces you to a classic: grilled chicken souvlaki with a side of quinoa and a Greek salad. The combination of lean protein, whole grains, and veggies will transport your taste buds to the shores of the Aegean Sea.

Day 4: Flavorful Fusion

Let's mix it up a bit today. Start your morning with a tropical smoothie – blend together some spinach, pineapple, banana, and coconut water. It's a nutrient-packed concoction that's as refreshing as it is healthy.

Lunch is a Mexican-inspired bowl with black beans, grilled chicken, avocado, and brown rice. Top it off with a squeeze of lime and a sprinkle of cilantro for that extra kick.

Dinner gets adventurous with a Thai-inspired shrimp stir-fry. Load it up with colorful veggies, toss in some cashews, and serve it over cauliflower rice. It's a low-carb option that doesn't compromise on flavor.

Day 5: Comfort Food, Elevated

Who says comfort food can't be healthy? Start your day with a bowl of oatmeal topped with sliced bananas and a dollop of almond butter. It's a warm and cozy breakfast that won't send your blood sugar on a rollercoaster.

Lunch brings a classic – a turkey and vegetable soup. Packed with nutrients, this bowl of goodness is not only delicious but also incredibly satisfying. Add a side of whole-grain crackers for that extra crunch.

Dinner tonight is a revamped favorite: spaghetti squash with turkey meatballs and marinara sauce. It's a low-carb alternative to traditional pasta, but the flavors are just as comforting.

Day 6: Quick and Easy

For a busy morning, whip up a quick green smoothie with kale, banana, and a splash of almond milk. It's a speedy, nutrient-rich option that ensures you start your day on the right foot.

Lunch features a tuna salad with mixed greens, cherry tomatoes, and a vinaigrette dressing. It's light yet satisfying, providing a good balance of proteins and greens.

Dinner keeps things simple yet delicious – grilled fish tacos with cabbage slaw and a squeeze of lime. Opt for whole-grain tortillas for that extra fiber kick.

Day 7: Celebrate Your Success

Congrats, you've made it to day seven! Breakfast is celebrated with a colorful fruit salad – a medley of your favorite fruits with a sprinkle of chia seeds for added texture and nutrition.

Lunch is a hearty and satisfying quinoa and black bean bowl. Load it up with veggies, avocado, and a drizzle of your favorite dressing.

Dinner wraps up the week with a lean beef and vegetable stir-fry. Serve it over a bed of cauliflower rice for a low-carb option that doesn't skimp on flavor.

Remember, each day is a step toward a healthier, more balanced you. Keep experimenting with flavors and ingredients, and let your taste buds guide you on this delicious journey!